T0349410

RADICAL REST

RADICAL REST

Notes on burnout, healing and hopeful futures

EVIE MUIR

Elliott&Thompson

First published 2024 by
Elliott and Thompson Limited
2 John Street
London WC1N 2ES
www.eandtbooks.com

ISBN: 978-1-78396-765-0

Copyright © Evie Muir 2024

The Author has asserted her rights under the Copyright, Designs and Patents
Act, 1988, to be identified as Author of this Work.

All rights reserved. No part of this publication may be reproduced, stored in or
introduced into a retrieval system, or transmitted, in any form, or by any means
(electronic, mechanical, photocopying, recording or otherwise) without the prior
written permission of the publisher. Any person who does any unauthorized
act in relation to this publication may be liable to criminal prosecution and civil
claims for damages.

Every effort has been made to trace copyright holders for material used within
this book. Where this has not been possible, the publisher will be happy to credit
them in future editions.

Permissions:
Page 187: Aurora Levins Morales, excerpt from 'V'ahavta'. Copyright © 2016 by
Aurora Levins Morales. Used with the permission of The Permissions Company,
LLC on behalf of Aurora Levins Morales, www.auroralevinsmorales.com

9 8 7 6 5 4 3 2 1

A catalogue record for this book is available from
the British Library.

Typesetting: Marie Doherty
Printed by CPI Group (UK) Ltd, Croydon, CR0 4YY

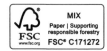

To my family:
Mum, Keith, Sam, Bradley, Jessie.

Extended family:
All the survivors daring to dream of, and fight
for, something beyond suffering.
More-than-human kin.

And the little girl who, when asked 'What do you want
to be when you grow up?' answered: 'An author'.

This is for you.

Contents

Notes on Language

Being from the North of England, I tend to have a playful approach to language. Up North we're not raised to speak the 'Queen's English' and I love that about us, and for us. Our turns of phrases, our commitment to omitting 'the' from our speech, our many terms of endearment with just as many colourful expletives: the way words form in a Northern mouth makes my heart sing.

Being an organiser in Black community spaces, on the other hand, has taught me that language is also something that should be taken seriously. It has the power to hurt and heal, to hide and bring to light, to erase and to platform, to appropriate and appreciate, to weaponise and mobilise. Our communities are lyricists. And we are constantly creating expansive terminology to articulate our suffering, express our joy and communicate our dreams.

Being a Black Northern writer and organiser therefore comes with its challenges. Holding both the complexities and creativity of the written word is one of them. I hope to do this here, by referring to some terms used within *Radical Rest* whose meanings are as important as they are evolving.

On 'Radical'

The Combahee River Collective, a Black Feminist collective based in the USA, remind us that 'if Black women were free, it would mean that everyone else would have to be free, since our freedom would necessitate the destruction of all systems of oppression.'[1]

Similarly, the UK-based author of *The Transgender Issue*, Shon Faye, states that 'the liberation of trans people would improve the lives of everyone in society'.[2]

What has always drawn me to Black Feminism as a political praxis is the ways it not only gives us language to articulate the conditions of our current reality but also offers the tools to ensure the liberation of all those oppressed.

To echo Lola Olufemi, 'I feel embarrassed when I say *feminism* and people do not think *revolution in service of every living thing*. I think I will spend my life trying to rectify this.'[3]

So, let me be clear. *Radical Rest* uses the term 'radical' in the context of this Black Feminist, futurist, liberatory legacy, not as a warped manipulative tool of fascism that prefixes 'trans-exclusionary'. This means that those most marginalised by society are not silenced in these pages, nor is our interdependent struggle with the more-than-human overlooked (the natural world and every living thing in it). After all, it is not just us mere humans who are burning out, but our environments too. If your feminism advocates for the subjugation and oppression of any community, you will not find your views represented here.

On 'Race'

It seems to me that all the terminology used to describe racial identity sits on a spectrum between imperfect and inadequate. *Radical Rest* is situated in the understanding that race is a social construct imposed through dominant hierarchies, which for some translates to individual and collective experiences of harm and oppression, and for others translates to power and privilege. With an intersectional recognition that this is never as one-dimensional as it may appear, I use language like 'people of colour', 'racialised communities' and 'global majority peoples' to describe all who, due to their race, fall into the former categorisation. In using these terms, I hope it is easier for readers to self-identify and centre their own experiences, but it is with an acknowledgement that some terms are more flawed than others. 'People of colour', for example, has rightfully been critiqued due to its proximity to 'coloured', and it is my prediction that it will become as redundant as 'BAME' (*ick*), and 'non-white' (*shudders*) in future years. As Suhaiymah Manzoor-Khan writes in *Seeing for Ourselves and Even Stranger Possibilities*: 'We rarely consider that instead of naming ourselves in relation to white supremacy, we could name white supremacy itself'.[4] Whilst *Radical Rest* intends to contribute to such a naming, I too have found the existing linguistic limitations challenging to overcome. It appears that a term that doesn't homogenise, minimise, distract or offend does not yet exist − I hope one day that it does.

I come to *Radical Rest* conscious of the duality of my privilege and dis-privilege: as a mixed-race person who is racialised as Black-but-not-quite. As a working-class person raised by a single parent on benefits in the North of England, who − despite having a fluctuating relationship with the benefits system myself − has also benefitted from formal education and academia. As someone who has suffered with disabilities that are lifelong and chronic, yet invisible, and therefore is arguably able to navigate society, and access care and community with greater ease than those with visible disabilities. And as someone who has been gifted the privilege and responsibility of being able to write a book in a world which systematically silences our words, despite the dis-privileges of the publishing industry that I have felt viscerally throughout the process of writing *Radical Rest* (thank you to Abi and Sarah for holding my hand along the way).

On 'Queer'

I also recognise my privilege and dis-privilege as someone who identifies with the expansive, undefining potential of queerness without having grown up in a generation where 'queer' was a life-threatening slur. Although 'queer' has experienced somewhat of a reclamation and resurgence in recent years, there are many who are understandably unable to embrace the term, due to its association with interpersonal and institutional oppression.

Just as language around race is regularly debated, I recognise the imperfections of language around gender and sexuality. I shy away from using LGBTQIA+ mostly due to personal preference. Although it remains extremely useful for individual self-identification and collective solidarity, there is an emerging recognition of the limitations of categorisation, and that the acronym is becoming as institutionally manipulated as, for example, BAME.

Throughout *Radical Rest*, therefore, I refer to 'queerness' in the hopes of capturing the breadth and depth of existence beyond the binaries of cis-hetero-normativity, and that those who understand themselves to be more expansive, more undefinable than society would like us to be, can see themselves in these pages.

On 'Abolition'

Throughout *Radical Rest* I talk of abolition as the long-standing fight against the prison industrial complex. My own introduction to abolitionist, anti-carceral politics comes from lived experience: as a survivor of domestic abuse who attempted and ultimately failed to navigate the so-called 'criminal justice system' in search of help and healing; and as a practitioner within the Violence Against Women and Girls (VAWG) sector who witnessed others similarly try, fail and emerge more harmed than before.

Though there is much to be talked about in relation to burnout and the prison industrial complex as an institution, it is through the abolitionist legacy of imagining a world without prisons that *Radical Rest* imagines a world without burnout. 'Racial Justice' therefore is referred to through the application of practices of worldbuilding, futurism and radical imagining – not through reformist policies such as 'diversity, equality and inclusion' (*bleurgh*).

Content Warning

Please note that *Radical Rest* contains references to suicide, suicidal ideation, self-harm, substance abuse, domestic abuse and sexual violence, racism and racial violence, institutionalisation, and police violence. To begin to heal from burnout requires self-exploration and self-reflection. This may be uncomfortable and may incite an emotional or physical response. Please do what you need to do to look after yourself and each other as you read this book.

Introduction

There is no end
To what a living world
Will demand of you[1]

Saturday, 20 July 2024

Today is the day in which the future begins for Lauren Olamina, the main protagonist in Octavia E. Butler's *Parable of the Sower* and, serendipitously, the same month and year that the book you have in your hands, *Radical Rest*, enters the world for the first time. First published in 1993, Butler's speculative fiction considers what the present-future of today may hold for a Black teenage girl growing up in the American South, or, that is, the remnants of it. Journeying through Lauren's formative years, this present-future is set within an apocalyptic landscape. Climate, economic and social crises amid political abandonment have led to deepening poverty, festering disease, rampant homelessness, indentured slavery, as well as widespread murder and robbery, and drug addiction as a means of survival. In Butler's 2024, nobody, not even the privileged – especially the privileged – is safe.

Though Butler's predictions may have been only *slightly* more damning than our Western realities – with people being forced to rob and kill each other for the little fruit that still grows in back gardens, and where scores of vigilantes, addicted to a new substance nicknamed 'pyro', burn every remnant of civilisation

– the eerie similarities in the ways society continues to fracture are undeniable.

Despite our own feverish avoidance of its ongoing nature, we have not long since emerged from the dazed remnants of a global pandemic. We now find ourselves amid an economic crisis where the cost of living is rising beyond our ability to meet our needs, while our world leaders continue to play with the rights and health of the planet and its most marginalised populations, as if our futures are nothing more than an egotistical game of monopoly. Meanwhile, as the days unfold, we are bearing witness to seemingly never-ending atrocities, with fascist imperialism setting the backdrop for the killing of Palestinian, Sudanese, Congolese and Haitian people.

That we are experiencing burnout in the face of such imminent catastrophe is not surprising. In fact, one could argue that burnout is the only logical response to the palpable powerlessness felt under racial capitalism – the dominant economic system under which we live. Ruth Wilson Gilmore, the prison abolitionist and scholar, states that 'capitalism requires inequality and racism enshrines it'. Under racial capitalism the individual is viewed as nothing more than a means of production, with impoverished, racialised and marginalised communities' labour disproportionately exploited. Within such a system, our emotional, physical and environmental health is at best something to be manipulated to serve capitalism, and at worst, completely ignored. That we are experiencing a widespread burnout is simply a symptom of a deeply sick society, and a signal that change is needed. 'We can't undo racism without undoing capitalism,' Gilmore says.

Despite being published thirty years ago, *Parable of the Sower* continues to be a mirror held up to the crumbling façade of this white, Western, capitalist society. And in many ways it serves as a spine-chilling projection of what may still be if our only relationship to every living thing continues to be one of merciless extraction. 'Those nightmares of mine are our future if we fail one another,' Lauren journals.[2]

Thursday, 26 March 2020

The Covid-19 pandemic should have been our call to arms. It should have been an opportunity for change, a real questioning of the ways our global and local communities had been operating, and an invitation to develop a society that is both safe and hospitable for people and planet. The Covid-19 pandemic should have turned us all into activists. For the first time we were collectively experiencing a lack of freedom, a lack of choice, a lack of control. Those who had once been protected by power and privilege were – at least temporarily – forced to get a glimpse of what it's like to exist on the margins of society, to be policed by the state, have your freedoms removed, have your choice and agency limited.

This should have instilled empathy and understanding for those who experience these oppressions as a part of everyday life, a moment to say, 'hang on a minute, nobody should be subjected to this'. Rather than fostering deeper love for and solidarity with one another, however, we simply became defined by grief and fear. Scared, bereft and overwhelmed, we deserved time to recover, process and rebuild. And from this healing, the opportunity for radical resistance could have been born. Instead? The UK and so many other countries rushed for a return to normalcy, and this denied us the opportunity for transformation. We were not permitted the space to question whether 'normal' was actually that great. Whether a society that creates the capacity for endless crises is functioning after all. What could have become a mobilised community became a collection of zombified individuals, expected to maintain our productivity and output while becoming increasingly socially isolated. What remains is a burnt-out nation.

Reflecting on the crisis of imagination and the limitations of reformist politics after a conversation with a childhood friend who just wants things to go back to how they were, Lauren writes 'she wants a future she can understand and depend on – a future that looks a lot like her parents' present. I don't think that's possible. Things are changing too much, too fast.'[3] She recognises that the society they once knew in *Parable of the Sower* – the society we now have – has never been an ideal. It serves some, but not all of us. She sees the potential in collapse, and despite all the horrors around her, remains steadfast in her belief that building something new is possible. 'It took a plague to make some of the people realise that things *could* change' she writes,[4] and in our own post-pandemic present, we are witnessing moments where these shifts are taking place, despite the drive from elsewhere to keep pushing onwards ever faster.

What has been termed 'The Great Resignation' is a prime example of this. An estimated 4 million workers quit their jobs in the UK following the home-working and public health measures during the pandemic. In its aftermath, almost 2.5 million public-sector workers went on strike, with healthcare, transport, education and the civil service experiencing intense disruption. Similarly, in the USA, the Bureau of Labor Statistics quantify that 47 million people left their jobs in 2021, with 50 million more following suit in 2022.

This professional re-evaluation of priorities and demand for greater employment rights represents a deep dissatisfaction with the ways capitalism expects employees to live and breathe their work for little to no return. Social media trends also offer an insight into a fast-spreading anti-capitalist consciousness, with 'soft life', 'bed rotting' and 'quiet quitting' signifying an appetite for change, and a yearning for purpose, pleasure and pause.

Despite these small indicators that we are becoming increasingly fed up with the status quo, we're now collectively running on empty amid a cost-of-living crisis and a callous expectation that we maintain our usefulness without even the guaranteed return of our basic needs being met. We're disenfranchised and resentful, weary and depressed, drained by the daily atrocities on the news and from feeling perpetually heavy after two years of hypervigilance, health anxiety and fear. With no opportunity to process these emotions, they are rendering us numb and inactive, too exhausted to revolt. Burnt out.

Though the few research papers that have examined the condition have only done so through the lens of 'occupational stress', studies into the physical and emotional effects of burnout have proven that it causes cognitive impairment, affecting the limbic structures,[5] the hippocampus (which stores information and converts experiences into memories), the amygdala[6] (which acts as our brain's emotional computer and alarm system) and the prefrontal cortex[7] (the part of our brain responsible for making rational decisions, upholding socially appropriate behaviour and understanding complex information). It also impacts the brain tissue in areas such as the caudate (which performs critical functions such as motor control, cognition and emotion), putamen volumes[8] (which oversee our learning and motor control, including speech articulation, language functions, reward, cognitive functioning and addiction) and cortisol levels[9] (which, when high, have drastic impacts on our stress levels). When impaired in some way, all of these areas of the brain influence a person's ability to modulate and regulate stressful or negative emotions.

Based on these findings, many neurologists surmise that the brain responds to burnout in almost identical ways as it does trauma, and that neurological symptoms of burnout mimic those associated with post-traumatic stress disorder (PTSD). It's for these reasons that many go as far as to advocate for burnout to be classified as a chronic illness, and that a trauma-informed approach to burnout is required. Treating burnout symptoms in the same ways that we do mere stress, it is reasoned, will not go far enough in rehabilitating the long-term effects.

To understand burnout through a trauma-informed lens, however, requires us to understand how our brains and bodies react to a traumatic event. When our amygdala is functioning correctly, for example, we have greater capacity to cope with everyday stresses. Under normal circumstances, our capacity to negotiate and navigate issues is larger and we can adequately assess and respond to situations. However, when we experience trauma, our window of tolerance shrinks dramatically, meaning the situations that once felt safe and comfortable to us are limited. Everything is perceived as threatening, and our brain responds accordingly.

Four of the more commonly recognised types of trauma responses include: fight mode – feeling the need to defend and protect yourself, with a person becoming angry, anxious, defensive or aggressive; flight mode – the desire to a flee a situation that we perceive to be threatening, through running away, impulsive actions or obsessive thoughts; freeze mode – the human equivalent of 'playing dead' with the inability to think or act in a moment, with forms including disassociation, shutting down, memory loss, feelings of being on autopilot; and fawn mode – the instinct to befriend your attacker to keep you safe. This is often controversially exemplified through 'Stockholm's Syndrome', but can also manifest through people pleasing, avoiding conflict and self-betrayal.

When our brains go into survival mode after we experience a traumatic event and these trauma responses become active to protect us, our brain is simply operating in this way to keep us safe within the moment. After the traumatic event, however, we can find that we're stuck in this state of hypervigilance because our brains have not identified that we are safe. This can have a long-term effect on how we perceive and interact with the world. Unsafe situations may feel comfortable, non-threatening situations may now be perceived as threatening, and our memories start to be stored incorrectly. This causes us to interact with people differently, exhibit risk-seeking behaviour, make irrational decisions and be vulnerable to further exploitation.

These trauma responses are not simply situated in our brains however, they represent a full-body response, guided by our nervous systems which absorb information through our senses, then process this information and direct our physiological reactions accordingly. Fundamentally, this means when we are burnt out, we are operating at the same levels of hypersensitivity and hypervigilance as we would had we experienced a traumatic event. The burnt-out body now assesses and responds to everyday workplace activities – challenging meetings, appraisals and progress reviews, office environments, mounting workloads or changes in responsibilities – as a genuine danger.

Understanding burnout in this way means its debilitating impacts can no longer be undermined as an unfortunate yet inconsequential side effect of work. It also means that at the individual level we can understand that we are, in fact, navigating labour through a constant exhibiting of trauma responses. We see that not only is work under capitalism traumatic, but present-day responses to burnout are inadequate, negligent to the point of perversion. And, while long-term support for trauma survivors of any kind is woefully undervalued and underfunded in the UK, if we wouldn't send a car crash survivor back inside their fiery vehicle, if we wouldn't advise a domestic abuse survivor to return to their abuser, if we wouldn't walk an assault survivor back to the site of their attack, why would we suggest that all a survivor of workplace trauma needs is a week off on sick leave to then return to their harmful place of employment?

If PTSD suggests that our trauma is situated in the past, perhaps burnout can be how we move away from pathologisation, to simply naming the traumas we experience that are present and ongoing; those which transcend the linear boundaries of the institutional and collide with the traumas of existing within a racial capitalist society. Understanding burnout through a trauma-informed lens, means a recognition that when we burn out, we seldom burn out equally. In centring 'activist burnout' in these pages, I am attempting to name the embodied trauma response that sits on the intersection of trying to exist with dignity and safety under white supremacy, patriarchy, ableism, islamophobia, homophobia and transphobia, while simultaneously resisting and reimagining these oppressions. It is the self-combusting exhaustion that arises when you care so much about society, within a society that doesn't care back. And, with our aliveness being dependent upon its success, it is impossible for those of us in movement spaces to separate ourselves from the work. This, I believe, is where we burn out. And, unlike a capitalist workplace which thrives on the disposability of its workers, when we burn out our movements die with us, and change ceases possibility. Though through a trauma-informed lens we can recognise the depth and scale of harm shouldered by people of colour, this does not make us helpless victims in need of saving; what it does mean is that we are the experts in our own salvation.

Our societies are failing so many of us under the disintegrating pillars that hold it aloft. Yet what might fill the place of this crumbling civilisation? And how might we build a burnout-free future from its remains? Here, we can look to the ideas that underpin abolition as our tools. Deeply rooted within the eradication of the prison industrial complex, abolition envisions and strategises for the elimination of imprisonment, policing and surveillance by creating structural alternatives to punishment and accountability. While the process of tearing down oppressive institutions is a fundamental factor, abolition asks for more than just demolition. It calls for the complete dismantling of the world as we know it and the building of a new one, one which will offer such an abundance of care that there will be no space in our minds, let alone our communities, for things like prisons. And it is here that abolition becomes the work of creating a world full of love, health, education, food, shared abundance, dignity, safety, justice, freedom and rest.

Abolition reminds us that it would be simply inefficient to look for solutions to burnout under racial capitalism – the place in which it thrives. As Gilmore assures, 'abolition is not *absence*, it is *presence*. What the world will become already exists in fragments and pieces, experiments, and possibilities. So those who feel in their gut deep anxiety that abolition means knock it all down, scorch the earth and start something new, let that go. Abolition is building the future from the present, in all of the ways we can.'[10]

When we create a landscape that no longer harms those most impacted by such systems of oppression, we will *all* benefit. It's for this reason that throughout *Radical Rest* you'll find the lived experiences of activists with intersectional identities centred, those who endure intersecting forms of oppression, both at the hands of our employers and the state. These are the activists, artists, organisers, movement builders, community leaders, frontline workers, healers and disrupters across the UK, who I consider co-conspirators and comrades. Those who I admire and who I am fortunate to do this work alongside of and because of.

I centre activists' experiences in these pages because although harm under capitalism may be inevitable regardless of your proximity to it, there are those who, I believe, are disproportionately impacted by burnout. A US study, for example, found that up to 50 per cent of activists have experienced burnout, 87 per cent of whom had to quit their activism within six years as a result.[11] Those who aren't activists may experience burnout, but for different reasons and in different ways. Namely, a corporate burnout can be understood as being deeply enmeshed *with* capitalism, rather than being marginalised from it. While the conditions of working under racial capitalism are likely to be traumatising for anyone, in a corporate workplace burnout is unlikely to be predetermined by intergenerational trauma – the emotional, physical, behavioural and genetic ways trauma is carried through generations – by working within your trauma, or having your trauma exploited as a condition of your employment.

A proximity to capitalism also offers an array of neoliberal benefits that provide the opportunity to rest. Material and financial security, social status and the additional accessibility of individualised wellbeing experiences, such as spa days or expensive wellness retreats, for example, alleviate the impacts of burnout and facilitate a swift return to the labour market to complete the whole cycle again. For activists, however, our positionality of being in resistance to these systematic oppressions means that we are also less likely to benefit from such offerings. Our work can't neatly fit into a nine-to-five window, and it's not something we can simply quit or take leave from like a statutory job. This work demands of us our capacity to be responsive, reactive, adaptable and malleable at all hours of the day. Beyond the boundaries of what is paid, our organising includes the unpaid and under-resourced emotional labour of supporting our communities, healing our traumas, advocating for our rights, and being responsive in our protests and campaigns when escalated action is required.

Similarly, rest – for activists – is more than simply having a break from capitalism in order to return to it later, nor is it the ease we associate with a privileged upper class. In many ways, our rest *isn't* radical at all. It is no more than a metabolic, psychological and spiritual need that is necessary for a healthy, meaningful existence. And yet, rest – as we'll come to see together as this book unfolds – is also the embodied healing of our pre-existing traumas. Rest is the space and time to reconnect with ourselves, our communities and the land. Rest is the ability to imagine, dream, create and build a future where burnout doesn't exist. To rest in this way, under racial capitalism, can only be an act of resistance.

Thursday, 10 May 2018

The ongoing trauma of living in a state of constant survival is something all too familiar for Lauren in *Parable of the Sower*, who is simultaneously plagued by her own embodied traumas. She was born with a condition called 'hyper-empathy syndrome', a side effect of her mother's prescription drug use during pregnancy. Those with hyper-empathy (often self-described as 'feelers' or 'sharers') feel what others feel. Every ache and pain, scrape and bruise, wound, internal or external.

Lauren describes the condition as an empathetic agony, which causes her bones to ache, her skin to bleed, her body to bruise as the relentless vibrations of others' pain seep into her core. Dissociative, detached and disembodied, she experiences the wounds of the injured, the decay of the barely living and the life fading from the dying. But does not die herself.

Like Lauren, I too have been plagued with (and this doesn't feel dramatic, or an exaggeration) the curse of being empathetically at the behest of my emotions. When I was twenty-four, I was diagnosed with borderline personality disorder while sectioned under the Mental Health Act in an institute in Rotherham. When the psychiatrist – a tall, white, balding man who was incapable of maintaining eye contact with me or any other inpatient there – issued this diagnosis, I rolled my eyes with boredom. *You sir, are at least a decade late.*

I had self-diagnosed myself with the condition before I'd even reached my teen years, thanks to the watching and rewatching and rewatching of *Girl, Interrupted*. In one scene, Winona Ryder's sparrow-like character, Susanna Kaysen, breaks into the doctor's office and steals her medical files. She reads the symptoms aloud to a captivated audience of fellow inpatients, describing the ways those with the condition are stereotyped to have an instability of self-image, relationships and mood, uncertainty about goals, impulsive in activities that are self-damaging, such as casual sex, social contrariness and a general pessimistic attitude. While having a name for the torment I was experiencing was, in many ways a comfort, when Susanna's fellow inpatients dismiss the diagnosis, it made me question whether I'm so abnormal after all.

Of course, no respectable medical professional (and when I was younger I saw many and varied) wanted to label a child with such a diagnosis. So, instead, I went undiagnosed and untreated – or at the very least, inadequately treated – for most of my childhood. Those big emotions and desperate coping mechanisms deepened alongside other unaddressed traumas and seismic griefs. I tried, and I imagine regularly failed, to maintain the façade of a normal teenager, but behind the scenes I was losing myself.

I now reject much of the alphabet spaghetti of diagnoses I've accumulated in my thirty years, and all the problematic, disproportionately gendered, racialised stigmas that come with them: BPD now emotionally unstable personality disorder (EUPD); PTSD upgraded to complex PTSD, or C-PTSD (complex only in the Western inability to offer support), PME, or PMDD (depending on how informed the medical professional is); anxiety disorder; depressive disorder – the list goes on. All of this is simply to say, I have big feelings. Huge feelings. Deep feelings. And these big, huge, deep feelings oftentimes dominate my life in a society that thrives on our disembodied, emotional suppression, and which keeps us preoccupied with pathologisation and individualistic forms of care.

Monday, 18 April 2005

As Audre Lorde once self-described, 'I was a mess. I was introverted. Hypersensitive. I was all of too intense. All of the words that other people use for little wild Black girls.'[12] Without healthy coping mechanisms amid so much emotional turmoil, I turned to self-harm in its many self-destructive forms and every adult around me panicked. What started as a quiet attempt at trying to release the pain through the razor-made crevices of my skin, thrust me into a scrutinised spotlight that I didn't want or need. My mum, teachers, social workers, GPs, child psychiatrists, parents of friends were all terrified of a child they deemed to be a danger to herself and others.

Somewhere between high doses of antidepressants (where side effects included 'suicidal thoughts'), hospitalisation and not feeling like I was allowed any moment to escape the pain in my brain, I found myself succumbing to suicidal ideation.

I often look back at those teenage years and can't help but feel sorry for that person – 'me', but not quite. It's a me I'm detached from, disassociated from. Me, but only in other people's memories, never my own. That version of me grew up a mixed-race Black girl, in a predominantly white, extremely working-class, ex-industrial area of Doncaster – the kind of town where dreams go to die or are moulded into a functional version of a dream that serves capitalism. A town that once boasted a bright purple UKIP coffee shop, where bigots could bond over tea, cake and their hatred of migration. A town where you surrounded yourself with people – often the wrong people – to distract yourself from the loneliness that never quietens. A town where leaving feels like an escape and returning incites nausea.

In Doncaster I grew up a cliché of unbelonging; fitting in as a teenager while navigating the static electricity of trauma felt impossible. Most of my school friends were years away from ever experiencing poor mental health. Very few had experienced a loss, none of them had ever lost themselves. And so, I held people at arm's length, not wanting anyone to come too close in case their hair stood on end, or they left singed. *You mustn't let them realise you're not normal*, I thought.

With her father recognising it to be a vulnerability that could be so easily exploited, Lauren's hyper-empathy is also seen as something to fear. I too have had more experiences than I thought I could endure where my vulnerability was manipulated. Too submerged in grief, unable to find a sense of self that could harness me to any stability, the arms of older, opportunistic men felt like safety. Under the guise of a 'relationship', these white men saw a vulnerable Black girl as something to abuse, fetishise and control. My first abusive relationship ensured my adolescent years were defined by stalking, harassment and strangling. When he tired of me was I able to leave him.

Bruised and broken, a second consecutive abusive relationship soon followed with a person who, over the course of six years, would proudly boast 'I've never hit you'. Too clever to ever leave a physical mark, his power was harnessed through the ability to reduce any sense of self, agency or identity to a malleable pile of jelly. A truly narcissistic person who has left scores of wounded women – no, girls – alongside me in his wake, he would then mould you into an obedient partner. One who could withstand whatever emotional torture he inflicted – the cheating, the gaslighting, the financial abuse, the sexual violence. I endured it all. Now, even though I can't remember the days, weeks, months or years from that time coherently, I'm still left with the residual feelings that girl carried. That's why, throughout *Radical Rest* we will explore how an embodied practice must be at the heart of our revolution. We cannot heal, create or build when we're stuck in the trauma responses of survival mode, but through the honesty of somatic practice – connecting mind and body – we can honour our hurt, feel the interconnectedness of our experiences and shift the internalised oppression within ourselves.

$$\sim\!\bigcirc$$

In *Parables*, Lauren begins to reframe her once shameful ability to feel as a potential tool for change, a strength that if everyone possessed would prevent suffering and harm. As she becomes attuned to the ways her hyper-empathy gifts her with the power to safeguard herself and those around her, she reasons that no one who could feel the pain of others would be compelled to inflict it. Having been isolated in her hyper-empathy her whole life, she then begins to yearn for a community with shared lived experience, people she can live among in safety and solidarity.

Like Lauren, I too find myself interested in the ways my emotions – our emotions – can be a transformative tool for our liberation from burnout. Even though there are days when I still can't quite imagine a healed and rested version of myself, I now trust that it is possible. This hope is new and novel. I realise that the only way to actualise this kind of healing is to delve into the depths of the emotions, understand them, work through them, discard what no longer serves me and let go of the pain to make room for joy and rest. It's for these reasons that each chapter within *Radical Rest* centres around an emotion that I have come to associate with burnout.

The first four chapters – which focus on exhaustion, grief, anger and anxiety – unpack the ways in which so-called 'negative' emotions are political and how they can be transformed into a tool for change. The final four – abundance, joy, hope and rest – interrogate why we so often feel a lack of these positive emotions, and pose the possible futures that could be created if they too were harnessed as a revolutionary tool. These are by no means the only emotions that I could have examined. Love, awe, gratitude, calm, excitement, pride, for example, could have found a home here too. Fear, guilt, shame, apathy, envy, greed also come immediately to mind. And depression. It may seem strange to omit an emotion – a state of being – that has dominated so many of our experiences, of my own experience. But I reason that we can understand depression as an omnipresent feature of burnout, the culmination of all the above. By addressing their intricacies, we can begin to open the possibility for a depression-free, burnout-free existence.

You may also question whether some of those chosen feelings are even an emotion at all, and for that I ask you to indulge me a little as I ponder what it would be like if abundance or rest was in fact an emotion that we nurtured. In *Parables*, Lauren tells us that nothing but rest can ease our pain. Here we consider what could be if we were more often able (or enabled) to enter a state of being, feeling, seeing and knowing. If we could transcend the confinements of exploitation and suffering. When understood in this way, rest *is* an emotion that I most certainly want to feel more often.

To situate this emotional exploration in tangible, systemic grounding, throughout *Radical Rest* you will also find four case studies dotted among the chapters. They are: The Home, Education, The Charity Industrial Complex and The Health Sector. These are all institutions that we have been told are 'caring' as a default and, therefore, are often beyond critique in the public consciousness. In these case studies, however, we embark on a deep dive into how racial capitalism has transformed all four into institutions of harm, with great propensity to influence the burnout so many of us experience.

You'll notice too that the events I share in *Radical Rest* don't follow a linear timeline. This is because for those of us existing with trauma, the moments of our life are rarely remembered in a consecutive fashion. As someone whose emotions can fluctuate moment to moment, hour to hour, day to day, I know this to be true. So in an attempt to capture the ways in which it is possible to jump from the harrowing replaying of a day in the life of an abusive relationship, to the hopeful, heart-full moments of a walk in the Peak District, to the freezing sensation of grief and isolation, these emotive chapters offer anecdotes from my life as I associate them with embodied feeling, not in the order in which they took place. In centring the emotions that both drive and impact our work, what I hope to pose in these pages is the intimate ways our traumas can be a transformative tool for burnout recovery in all of us. The personal is, after all, political.

Sunday, 24 April 1932

From a feeling, an intuition, a need; from questions whose answers lie floating just out of reach, throughout *Parable of the Sower* we follow Lauren's evolving commitment to envisioning something other than the pain around her. As her observations become verses, verses become visions, and visions become a tangible plan and ethos in which to live by, 'Earthseed' is born in Lauren's imagination.

A religion? Perhaps. But only in that Lauren redefines God not as an omniscient power but as change. If God is change, Lauren reasons, then it is actually *we* who are the powerful, *we* who can incite change for good, *we* who can create a haven in which sharers – those who feel deeply – can thrive. What unfolds is the building of a community which, by virtue of her hyper-empathy, is a safe place to feel pain and let it go. Suppression, self-medication, self-mutilation and a commodified notion of self-care are all coping mechanisms that have allowed us to survive so far, Lauren realises, but sooner or later we must face these false promises of capitalism and transform them into something that can serve the community.

Upon realising the impossibility of accessing healing and justice in the Violence Against Women and Girls (VAWG) sector in which I once worked, I left in search of alternative possibilities for survivor's care, ones that also allowed me to heal alongside my community. Peaks of Colour is the humble manifestation of exactly that. A Peak District-based grassroots nature-for-healing community group, by and for people of colour only, Peaks of Colour exists as an informal yet intimate invitation for members of our community to join me on a journey of abolitionist imagination, nature-allied community care and healing justice. Through our walkshops – creative and holistic workshops in nature – we collaborate with other artists and activists of colour to curate spaces for those with gendered and racialised trauma.

I founded the group from a place of extreme burnout and as a result I was adamant that, in its initial form, a monthly walking club was all it would ever be. When I left the VAWG sector, however, I began to experience a gradual capaciousness. My ability to imagine strengthened, and with it Peaks of Colour's place and purpose in a broader movement for racial, gendered and land justice became firmly rooted in our local soil. Now, our work seeks to be a small, slow, soft revolution, whose home is in the rolling hills and leafy valleys of the Peak District.

Our restful rebellion is not the first that the Peak District's landscape has witnessed. The Kinder Mass Trespass, which took place in 1932, was a widespread protest that saw an estimated 400 working-class people from around Manchester and Sheffield convene across popular Peak District landscape, Kinder Scout. The march resisted the ways wealthy landowners forbade public access to the countryside and is credited with influencing the creation of UK national parks – the Peak District being the first – as we know them today.

That I should be drawn to a place with such radical history, in the moments when I was fleeing both an abusive relationship and oppressive workplace, now feels like an unconscious calling. Regular access to nature has been documented to substantially improve our physical and mental health and, over the years, and I have come to rely on the Peak District for my own trauma recovery as heavily as I do any other form of therapy. Like many artists, poets, writers, scientists and ecologists who have come before me, I am grateful to have the opportunity to experience the breathtaking promise of aliveness this place offers. Through Peaks of Colour, it is my hope that this journey does not have to be traversed alone, and that together we can grow a rested, mobilised movement.

Thursday, 17 August 2023

By now you may be thinking, 'I'm not an activist, this book's not for me'. Though I can't speak to the corporate experience in these pages, I hope it's possible for those whose work doesn't neatly align with that of 'activism' (in truth, there is very little neat about it) to still find some meaning, guidance, maybe even transformation here. That you do is vital in this fight for a restful revolution. After all, the responsibility of dismantling and deconstructing racial capitalism cannot lie solely with the oppressed without, once again, facilitating our inevitable burnout.

This fight requires those who benefit from such systems to reflect on their role in perpetuating harm and inequality, and to join us in active solidarity. While our lived experiences and our traumas may be disproportionate, we all share a mutual oppressor. Maybe in these pages you will find pause to reflect on the ways your participation in capitalism influences burnout in racialised communities, or perhaps you will be able to identify the ways your own strengths and skills can facilitate the movement. Either way, creating a society where rest isn't simply a break from dominant structures that is afforded to the privileged and powerful is a collective responsibility.

Perhaps this is also a good time to hold the complexities and contradictions of who is considered an activist. When we hear the word 'activist' we often think of those marching en masse on the front lines, megaphone in one hand and a placard in the other. There's an element of sacrifice and disruption associated with this imagined activist. Maybe they're chanting and screaming, tying themselves to lampposts, or on a hunger strike. This type of activism is known as 'direct action', and while it is an integral form of movement work, it is not the only role available to play.

But by positioning activism through this limiting lens, we exclude scores of people who, for a range of reasons, can't participate in this way, or who participate in other ways that are integral to successful action. Despite caring being central to their work, teachers and nurses, for example, are not considered activists in their day-to-day roles – unless, that is, they strike. As we saw in the days when the public health and cost-of-living crises merged, almost overnight striking public-sector employees went from being the nation's heroes who were clapped for in the height of the pandemic, to being demonised by the media and penalised by the state. Though their current proximity to systems of colonialism and capitalism often means we can't see the education and healthcare systems we currently have as sites of abolition, it's not difficult to imagine how transformative these institutions could be, if they were seen as opportunities for resistance, rather than merely a vocation. I write *Radical Rest* at a time when this binary notion of activism is being weaponised and criminalised by a Tory government. Amid a national campaign to disassociate the public from a sense of collective responsibility, that so many are yet to identify their place in the movement, or are afraid to consider themselves activists, is benefiting no one more than the state.

Deepa Iyer's 'Social Change Institution's Ecosystem Framework'[13] is a useful tool for mapping the multiple and varied roles we can all play in an anti-capitalist resistance to burnout. The roles offered within this include: the disrupter, the healer, the storyteller, the guide, the weaver, the experimenter, the front-line responder, the visionary, the builder and the caregiver, and they are all important and necessary components when creating meaningful change. This means that no matter who we are, we all have something personally and professionally to offer in the fight for social justice. The stay-at-home parent, the cleaner, the artist, the construction worker, the avid gardener, the tech-whiz, the daydreamer, the kid who's always in detention, the executive director, will all be able to see themselves within this framework. This is one of the things I find most encouraging – that alongside helping us to identify our own place within the movement, through the concept of an ecosystem we recognise that we are more effective, and our movements are more sustainable, when we align our efforts and distribute roles according to where we can thrive the most. This relinquishes the responsibility of a few people assuming all the roles, or roles we are less suited to, and burning out in the process.

Just as Peaks of Colour is a space in which we can experiment on the intersections of racial, gendered and land justice, *Radical Rest* is also a playground in which we can speculate. It's for this reason that if you came here for quick-fix solutions, answers, conclusions, advice or direction, you will likely be disappointed. You won't find a cure for burnout here either. I simply can't profess to have the answers. I am in the trenches with you, floundering against tidal waves of capitalism, and for the most part I rarely feel afloat. I too have felt on many occasions like I was drowning in a sea of over-whelm and overworkedness. And while Peaks of Colour has been my self-made raft with which to weather the storm, I haven't yet succeeded fully. In short, I'm still burnt out.

Radical Rest is, therefore, simply a modest attempt at seeking and sharing a lifeline. It is an invitation for you, the reader, to join me on my own ongoing journey of burnout recovery – one that seeks, with hope and sometimes desperation, to find alternatives to what is ultimately a dire situation. Despair, I find, sits in the acidic, belching stomach of acceptance. The possibility that this painfully exhausting life should be the only option for us is one I'm not yet prepared to yield to. These pages, therefore, are where we can consider the transformation required of our present and future and ask: how does it feel to be truly rested? What does a society look like in which we can rest? What do we need to dismantle and what do we need to build in order for our rest to be actualised?

There have been many moments during the course of writing *Radical Rest* when the answers to these questions have felt beyond my reach. There have also been questions posed to me that urged me to reckon with what I wanted this book to be. One such time was during an artists' residency hosted by RESOLVE Collective. Here I met André Anderson, fellow author and headmaster of the alternative art college Freedom & Balance, for the first time. I was introduced as someone writing their debut book on burnout, and without a moment's hesitation André said: 'Three questions immediately come to mind, if you don't mind me asking.'

'How are you writing this book without burning out yourself?'

'How are you writing this book in a way that ensures you will return to it yourself, if you were to experience burnout in the future?'

'How are you writing this book so that your readers don't burn out?'

My only answer to all three was: I wasn't. Alongside building a community group from the grassroots and trying to survive despite my own material insecurities within a cost-of-living crisis, I have reached burnout multiple times throughout the process of writing *Radical Rest*. Being transparent about this here, at the very beginning, feels necessary, not only to rid myself of the guilt-ridden reflex of imposter syndrome, but also to ground this exploration in the messy imperfections of its reality. Throughout, I have been reminded consistently that healing is hard and I have found the process of excavating my own traumas in order to examine and communicate them on these pages necessary but excruciating. I have become burnt out on the intersections of overthinking and under-being, and I've felt like a hypocrite and a failure for my inability to be emotionally present throughout. I carry a lot of guilt about this. I don't think I've been a very good partner, daughter, sister or friend during the process of writing this book, and upon the realisations prompted by André's questions, I felt like I was letting soon-to-be readers down by not being able to practise what I preach too.

When my emotions feel too overpowering to navigate, however, engaging with Black Feminist text returns me to a state of comfort and calm. When I need to better understand myself, the world and my place within it, I turn to Black Feminism and receive grounding and clarity. When I am feeling lost in this work, Black Feminism offers me direction and purpose. I am repeatedly awestruck by the way I find Black Feminist theory, or rather how it finds me, every time I need it the most. Black Feminism feels like a constant homecoming.

On one such day, I noticed that I was disassociating as I questioned, not for the first time, if finishing this book would be possible, safe even. I was numb, on autopilot, and reached for bell hooks' *Teaching to Transgress*. The pages flipped themselves to a pause, and my eyes rested on a previously highlighted quote towards the end of a page:

'It is not easy to name our pain, to theorise from that location.'[14]

To expose our wounds is a vulnerable undertaking, hooks reminds us, but to do so facilitates our remembering and recovering of ourselves and renews a commitment to liberation. From this self-excavation we can transform the trauma within into healing words, healing strategies, healing theory.

It is in this Black Feminist tradition of speaking lived experience into theory, and theory into practice, that Octavia E. Butler captures so seamlessly in her *Parables* series. This is what *Radical Rest* seeks, humbly and with gratitude, to honour in these pages. This process of cultivating a racial imagination from pain and pedagogy, however, is not without difficulty. The lows can still feel suffocating, and the healing process is rarely comfortable, yet through the burnout recovery journey in which *Radical Rest* is situated, I am, increasingly, hopeful. The provocation is that together we can begin to identify the traumas we carry deep in our bones, name the ways our burnout manifests within racial capitalism and recognise the depth of impact that this has on us as individuals and as a society. From this self-knowing, we can begin a journey of collective repair. And in this healing of ourselves, each other and the land, deepen our understanding of our purpose in creating this change. *Radical Rest* posits with optimistic assertion that there *can* be an end to oppression under racial capitalism, that burnout *can* be eradicated; that rest *can* be achieved. As Ruth Wilson Gilmore says: 'It's possible. It's really possible. And not in a romanticised way, but in a material, deliberate, consciousness exploding way. It's possible.'[15]

On Radical Exhaustion

When we set about trying to transform
society, we must remember that we
ourselves will also need to transform.
— Mariame Kaba[1]

For a mixed-race Black toddler growing up in the 1990s, watching old black and white Hollywood movies seems a peculiar pastime. Yet this was how I spent my childhood. While the Disney Channel and Nickelodeon entertained my peers, I sat cross-legged in front of the telly at my grandparents' two-up two-down terraced house and formed intimate connections with the likes of Cary Grant and Katharine Hepburn. With an Afro halo, impressionable eyes and an old soul, it was here that I developed a sense, though not yet an understanding, of the depths of my emotions. My grandma would often come into the living room to find me weeping, overwhelmed with empathy, moved by the swell of a saxophone or the romance of a just-lips-no-tongue kiss. The silver screen was the first place I saw people who looked like me: Lena Horne, Louis Armstrong, Sidney Poitier, Dorothy Dandridge. It was also where I first saw racism depicted in Technicolor, though I didn't have the vocabulary for it then. My face would contort into a question mark, trying to make sense of why so many roles portrayed by Black people were of inferiority and of the way those actors, such as Hattie McDaniel, were treated behind the scenes.

1

Exhaustion as The Blues

Alongside *The Wizard of Oz* – and later, *The Wiz* (my proudest moment as a child was playing Dorothy in my primary school's rendition) – one of my favourite films was *Show Boat*. I can't recall how deeply I understood their meaning, but at no more than five years old, the lyrics of 'Ol' Man River', sung by Paul Robeson, reverberated through my core. Through thick wet tears I would sing along, overwhelmed by how weary, sick of trying, tired of living and afraid of dying I also felt. Perhaps these lines resonated with a deep ancestral pain – maybe that's all empathy ever really is. Or perhaps their effect on me was a foreshadowing of the suicidal ideation that would consume me by the time I was twelve. Either way, the morbid toddler that I was declared that 'Ol' Man River' would be my funeral song. To this day, despite a critical under-standing of the song's problematic contexts and origins, I can't listen to it without crying. The kind where you feel the cracks in your heart widen with each pulsating crescendo.

With its depiction of a disregarded, weary workforce facing the physical exertion of relentless, thankless manual labour, 'Ol' Man River' flirts with a Black Marxist commentary on the exploit-ation of Black workers and our subsequent burnout. It's a song that reflects Robeson's own politics too, which supported civil rights and the Labour movement. Its lyrical pentatonic melody, along-side its deep messaging, situates it within the blues genre, whose lamenting, stretching notes, raspy, raw vocals and rhythmic, moody tempos espouses tiredness in so many of its songs.

The African American writer and critic Ralph Ellison calls the blues 'an impulse to keep the painful details and episodes of a brutal experience alive in one's aching consciousness, to finger its jagged grain, and to transcend it, not by the consolation of philoso-phy but by squeezing from it a near-tragic, near-comic lyricism.'[2]

2

Burnout, in the ways it exhausts us into a liminal state of awake-
ness, also feels like an aching consciousness. It's not the kind of
tiredness you feel after simply not getting enough sleep, but an
all-consuming, full-body depletion of energy. A world-weariness
that we drag with us, that weighs down in our bones and withers
our muscles. An exhaustion that makes you question whether you'll
ever feel energised again, that untethers you from your aliveness,
whispering daydreams of death as the only place you could ever
truly feel rested. Exhaustion, our theme for this chapter, is the
blues personified.

Insomnia has always been one of my most prominent trauma pres-
entations. When I'm struggling with my mental health, it's often
impossible for me to fall asleep. I need my partner safely beside me
for security, and when I eventually do drift off, I experience nightmares associated with specific traumas until I wake up at 7.30 a.m.
on the dot to resume my role as a well-trained cat mum reporting for breakfast duty. I rarely feel rested. Yet when I'm burnt
out, I find myself in the deepest of slumbers, resigned to my bed
for days. In this comatose state – from which I can rouse myself
only to use the toilet – preparing food and eating, maintaining
an acceptable level of personal hygiene and socialising (especially
socialising) all feel like unattainable tasks from a distant memory.

   I drift away from the version of myself I once knew in a cloud
of brain fog, unable to be present. My eyes stare wide and my
limbs feel like lofty appendages disconnected from my torso. My
body weighs heavy, enveloped in blankets of despair. Too absent to
even feel shame at my inactivity, the most stimulation I can mus-
ter is the comforting mumblings of a 'safe programme' (usually

radio adaptations of old Hollywood movies such as *It Happened One Night*). I hear their words, but I can't engage. This exhaustion can consume me for days, weeks at a time. A thick grey fog that vanishes me into a dissociative numbing space, empty of all feelings and sensations other than the need to simply lie down.

As lonely as this state of being feels, I know I'm not alone in my experiences. In fact, I barely know a single person who isn't also trying to claw themselves out of the depths of burnout. When we check in on each other, offering platitudes loaded with care but laced with the guilt of being too numb to do more for those we know are also suffering, the way we describe our current states is always the same: we're exhausted.

When I think of this type of exhaustion, I think of the painting *Blue Monday* by Annie Lee, which was created in 1985, almost sixty years after 'Ol' Man River' was released. *Blue Monday* is a self-portrait that depicts a faceless Black woman perched on the edge of a bed, head adorned with Bantu knots and bowed between her heightened, tensed shoulder blades. In the uninviting, tired environment that she inhabits, a calendar hangs on the wall behind her with a large 'X' signifying the day of the week. On the bedside table, the hands of an alarm clock tell us it's 5 a.m. These two items are the only indicators of what lies beyond the room. They suggest that as time passes, as the days merge into weeks and the weeks merge into months, this tired scene is repeated every morning, and that this weariness stays with this woman, even as she moves outside of these four walls.

Aside from the woman herself, and the subtle glow of yellow emanating from the bedside lamp, the painting is illustrated only in shades of blue. Her brown skin complements the blue's tonality, however, giving the impression that our woman is succumbing to the depression of a dreary room. The use of laboured, hopeless brushstrokes dragging their way down the page adds to this sense of her sinking heavily into the cold, dark, hollow anticipation of the day ahead.

Wearing a white nightgown, the subject is poised with one slipper on her foot and the other just out of arm's reach. Witnessing the way her hands support the weight of her body as she physically prepares herself to rise and emotionally prepares herself for the day ahead, I recognise all too well the waiting room of disassociation, where minutes feel like milliseconds. Time rushes by as you pause to inhale deep breaths and exhale weariness. *It'll fly by*, you reason. *Don't call in sick, you need the money*, you remind yourself. *Get up for, fuck's sake. You're gonna be late.* There's no time for self-compassion in these moments of motivation.

It's said that Lee, known for her realistic depictions of the everyday experiences of Black people, purposely omitted a face in *Blue Monday* in order to allow Black women in particular to relate to her work on a deeper level: 'I think my paintings connect me to women,' Lee says in an interview from 1997. 'I know that how I feel is the way a lot of women feel.'[5] I'm grateful for this creative decision. In *Blue Monday* I'm reminded of biting winter mornings, where seasonal depression compresses my skull. I can smell the freshness of the eerily tranquil pre-dawn air, and I can taste the sour-mouthed dryness that comes with the un-instinctual self-betrayal of denying my body the sleep it so desperately needs. Another – perhaps unintentional – effect of the facelessness of the subject is it makes us consider the lack of identity we're permitted to have within a system of regimented time – obedient workers all waking to begin our exhausted morning routines. Capitalism makes people faceless, and *Blue Monday* reminds us of this.

Despite the undeniably endless, escapeless pit of exhaustion that *Blue Monday* portrays, there's something about being able to see ourselves depicted in that weary state that's comforting. Not only does it allow us to feel less alone in this grind, but it wakes us up to the realisation that this life isn't healthy, that this feeling of dragging ourselves out of bed every morning shouldn't be the norm. A new generation of purveyors was given the opportunity to witness themselves in this way in 2022, when pop artist Lizzo paid homage to *Blue Monday* in a *Saturday Night Live* set designed to imitate the piece. Almost forty years after its creation, the painting still resonated with its audience. As one Twitter user shared: '*[Blue Monday]* hung in every Black household at the turn of the 21st Century. It fully encapsulates our mood today. We are beyond tired.'[4]

This exhaustion is both gendered and racialised. Over generations our communities have inherited a sleep deficit – the intended consequence of the theft of restorative sleep, which has been used as a tool to subjugate and extract labour from our communities for hundreds of years. In the mid-seventeenth century, African villages were raided at night so that people could be stolen into slavery, and squalid and cramped conditions on transatlantic vessels ensured slave quarters were completely incompatible with rest. On plantations, enslaved women were sexually assaulted by white men in their sleep. With the goal of slave masters being to 'keep the slave physically strong but psychologically weak [...] keep the body, take the mind',[5] rest became a punishable offence, warranting heightened surveillance. As the African American abolitionist and civil rights activist Frederick Douglass once wrote, 'more slaves are whipped for over-sleeping more than for any other fault'.[6] This extraction of sleep and labour did not stop with the abolition of slavery, however. It only morphed into the racist pseudoscience of eugenics, which – as we'll explore in depth in our case study on the health sector – subjected our communities to dehumanising medical tests so as to label Black communities as lazy and slow – racist stereotypes that still exist today.

Under racial capitalism as we now know it, contemporary conditions of sleep deprivation see racialised communities working disproportionately long hours in numerous, precarious, low-salaried, insecure or unstructured jobs. Shift work, zero-hours contracts and overtime are common. Also rife are physically and emotionally unsafe work environments where institutional racism dominates our experiences. After work, we're then more likely to return to overcrowded homes in noisy, polluted neighbourhoods, where deep, restorative rest is once again kept from us. This deliberate fragmentation from rest – which can be seen within every corner of society, from city planning to employee welfare – is not just life-altering, it's life-threatening. Breonna Taylor, a twenty-six-year-old African American woman who was killed in her sleep in 2020 when a team of plain-clothes police officers forced entry into her apartment during an unwarranted house raid, is evidence of this. When at rest, Black people continue to be regarded as loitering, trespassing, deviant, arrestable, unworthy of life.

Emerging research is capturing the ways in which the enduring legacy of this trauma is impacting our physical and mental health. In America, for example, one study concluded that Black people were five times more likely than white people to get less than six hours of sleep a night,[7] while Chinese participants were 2.3 times less likely, and Hispanic people were 1.8 times less likely. Meanwhile, a Centers for Disease Control and Prevention study on these 'racial and gendered sleep gaps' found that almost 50 per cent of all Black, Native Hawaiian, Pacific Islanders and Multiracial Americans achieved less than seven hours of sleep a night.[8]

While UK-based data is in short supply, the NHS estimates that one in three people suffer from poor sleep,[9] with a 2018 study finding that British adults get 8.76 days[10] less sleep a year than the global average. This significantly increases when examined through a gendered lens, with another study finding that the average woman loses forty-five days of sleep a year,[11] while another recognised that one in two British women[12] constantly feel sleep-deprived. A study looking at the 'ethnic differences in sleep duration' in the UK found that inadequate sleep was twice as prevalent in British Black people than in their white counterparts.[13] We're also documented to suffer from the highest rates of sleep disorders, such as insomnia or sleep apnoea, conditions which increase the risk of heart failure and coronary heart disease.[14]

When we understand the severity of the problem, suddenly the term 'staying woke' takes on a new meaning. This term acknowledges the struggles our ancestors faced and which we continue to face today, popularised through contemporary rhythm and blues songs such as Erykah Badu's 'Master Teacher' and Childish Gambino's 'Redbone'. This is a sleep epidemic. When closing our eyes poses a risk to life, remaining awake becomes a tool of hypervigilance – the only way to ensure our protection. Sayings such as 'I'll sleep when I'm dead' and 'sleep with one eye open' take on a far too sinister and literal interpretation as well. As communities across the globe continue to navigate complex social and historical relationships with sleep deprivation, this state of constant fatigue is used to break our resolve, keeping us compliant in our numbness.

Exhaustion as a Living Death

As racialised communities, we are expected to overextend ourselves so frequently that it becomes the norm. We're expected to exist as we oscillate in and out of this bodily breaking point, and often it is only when we're physically immobilised by burnout that we're able to name the exhaustion at all.

Vera Chapiro, community organiser and member of the artistic London-based Bare Minimum Collective,[15] defines burnout as a never-ending cycle of survival. Speaking to me over Zoom, she reflects that, 'We're often led to believe that burnout is a destination, and only when at that destination are we incited into action. But I think we're constantly in a continuum of differing degrees of burnout, never quite whole or healed.' She introduces me to the work of Martin O'Brien, a visual performance artist and scholar who was born with the chronic illness cystic fibrosis. Martin's art takes audiences on an exploration of mortality through physical endurance and pain-based practices in order to examine what it means to be born with a life-shortening disease, and to live longer than expected. In his series of performances *The Last Breath Society (Coughing Coffin)*, which was showcased at London's Institute of Contemporary Arts, O'Brien offers a living installation co-curated with 'sick queers, old queens and others thinking about death, who gather together, breathe together, mourn their lives and rehearse for the inevitable.'[16]

In interviews and biographies O'Brien describes himself as 'enjoying life as a zombie', something which Vera says really resonated with her and the Bare Minimum Collective. 'This idea of "Zombie Time", those of us who understand ourselves as in a state between life, living and some form of social, spiritual death. I think burnout can be put in that category, along that continuum. People often describe capitalism as a "death machine",' she says, 'but I understand capitalism as more of a machine that keeps us *just* alive enough to stay in or go back to work. And because what we need for living is made into profit, we all exist in conditions that drive us to this place of burnout.' In this context, our healthcare systems exist only to make sure we're healthy enough to work (or to be *declared* healthy enough to work).

That our state of burnout is often connected to the cultural phenomenon of 'the zombie' seems fitting, especially when considering Ruth Wilson Gilmore's definition of racism as 'the state-sanctioned and/or legal production and exploitation of group-differentiated vulnerabilities to premature death'.[17] Here we begin to see how everything from unaffordable housing and utilities to the incremental privatisation of healthcare and the ever-increasing age of retirement are interconnected geographies, constituting a web of state-manufactured precarity that robs us of our aliveness.

The 'living dead' caricature, now commonly associated with an escapist fantasy in horror movies, was actually coined as an African-Caribbean trope during the transatlantic slave trade.[18] In Haitian folklore, for example, the zombie archetype mirrored the inhumanity of the sleep-deprived slavery that existed there for over two centuries. In fear of being imprisoned in their enslaved bodies forever, slaves believed that the only way to escape their oppressive conditions was to die, returning to Africa in the after-life. Suicide, however, would condemn you to inhabit a soulless enslaved body for eternity, and the zombie became a representation of both existing realities and projected fears.

Like Gilmore, Achille Mbembe agrees that 'the function of racism is to regulate the distribution of death, and to make possible the murderous functions of the state'.[19] The historian and critical theorist, whose skill in holding the panoramic intricacies of colonialism and its legacies transcends multiple schools of thought, describes how racial oppression is still used as a state-sanctioned tool and is the ultimate expression of sovereignty – of state power. It 'resides to a large degree in the power and capacity to dictate who may live and who must die, mean[ing] the capacity to define who matters and who does not, who is disposable and who is not and which is expressed predominantly as the right to kill'.[20] The ways in which the state, as enforcers and upholders of racial capitalism, can be the architects of a life of suffering and survival or thriving and joy, encapsulates what Mbembe terms 'necropolitics'.

Necropolitics, Mbembe argues, captures how our contemporary societies are deployed as a weapon to create death-worlds – 'new and unique forms of social existence in which vast populations are subjected to conditions of life conferring upon them the status of *living dead*.'[21] Here, to be in a state of burnout is to exist in a kind of death-world, where you are not only incapable of functioning under the façade of racial capitalism, but are also unable to imagine a world free from it. In this death-world, rest is not only denied but replaced with the trauma of multiple forms of oppression. Burnt out by existing outside the privileges of whiteness, cisnormativity, ableness and heteronormativity, we're not only unable to actualise an affirming life, but we're also too burnt out to mobilise and revolt against an oppressive one.

Exhaustion as a Portal of Possibility

If I were to describe a death-world, the UK, at the time of writing this book, would encapsulate it perfectly. My generation, a demographic of late-twenties and early-thirties millennials, have lived through two recessions, a cost-of-living crisis, a global pandemic and decades of suffocating austerity. At a time in our lives when we should be thriving, frolicking, embracing the vast landscape of possibilities young adulthood has to offer, we're frantically worrying about the cost of bread, bills and how we're going to pay for the roof over our heads as our landlords mercilessly increase the rent. No longer able to access the rewards that a participation in capitalism guaranteed for our parents and grandparents (such as a foot on the property ladder or early retirement), our income has at best stagnated and at worst decreased, while inflation sees the cost of our basic needs soaring.

We're a depressed and anxious generation. In a supposedly post-pandemic world, we've become acutely aware of our mortality, unable to process the incomprehensible suffering we've witnessed. Death feels close, yet our once revolutionary health service is becoming increasingly privatised, with life-threatening waiting lists and services that range from the inaccessible to the traumatising. A nation that has perfected the art of cognitive dissonance, we embrace a political rhetoric of denial, desperate for a return to 'normal', even if 'normal' was itself shit. Everyone I know is practising, with relentless stamina, the British motto of 'Keep Calm and Carry On', suppressing the simmering anxiety of the next climate catastrophe, health crisis or oppressive government policy.

Nearly everyone I know is also medicated in some way, be that antidepressants, recreational drugs, alternative medicines or the inhalers that Vera and I wave at each other over Zoom. 'It's giving sickly Victorian child,' she laughs, before returning to a serious tone: 'Our bodies shouldn't be this worn down, so young. But I think they're reflecting the ills of the world. Capitalism makes us sick: diluted forms of death, diluted forms of sickness.'

In this context, it's never felt more important to search for and maintain thriving communities, vehicles in which to transport us through portals of possibility. As a result, more organisers are centring resistance to exhaustion as a core practice. The Bare Minimum Collective is one of them. A community of self-defined 'Black feminists, reluctant writers, artists, queer theorists, filmmakers, architects [...] who work across mediums with no regard for disciplinary boundaries', emerging from the University of

Cambridge, their manifesto is truly a feast for the eyes. It's cheeky, rebellious and deviant – they know the rules are arbitrary and ridiculous, and no one is going to convince them of their supposed relevance. Read aloud, their declaration of non-conformity feels like a sermon, spoken from a pulpit to a congregation of worn-out, exhausted bodies, starved of inspiration and thirsty for change. It describes the ethos that the collective wants to embody and espouse as mundane, yet not minimalist: worthless, directionless, wayward, lazy, yet creative and future-building. 'We're not interested in what will come of this,' they write. 'Maybe it will fail, we welcome failure! Call it a reaction to the boomers, a result of the financial crash, precarity, insecure housing, but every dream of stability has been shattered and we think that offers us something.'

Speaking on the collective's approach to forging alternatives, Vera tells me: 'Our understanding of art is something which makes each other and by extension another world possible. This really starts with facilitating ourselves. Art is a way of channelling our desire to live better, to sustain each other, to exist in relation, to find ways to thrive, when, every single day, it feels like we're confronted with the impossibility, or all the contradictions of life within a society that makes living seem impossible.' I notice her smiling as she says this, and we pause for a moment to discuss the shift in feeling – purpose, contentment, peace – that comes with submitting to the exhaustion and embracing the differences in being it offers. She continues, 'Our approach to our art is ad hoc and hodgepodge. We get together, are honest with each other about our levels of capacity, stress, fears. Our engagement fluctuates. We're all navigating our own problems, the housing crisis, grief, heartbreak. So many of us are living with intensifying forms of disability or chronic illness. So I'd say behind the scenes of Bare Minimum is the messiness of our interconnected lives. Then we carve out time and space and come as we are, and it's our excitement for change that fuels how we make new things happen.'

Their manifesto speaks to more than simply working on their own terms, however. There's a political commitment woven through their facetiousness too, daring readers to open their eyes and dream beyond a basic need for survival. It showcases an anticapitalist model of community care in action. On what it looks like to embody the ethos of the manifesto in everyday life, Vera says, 'We're giving ourselves permission to think of ways to not just *not* be dead, but also to really live.' I ask her how it feels to be part of a space that transports you to such freeing realities, and she pauses, nervously rubbing her palm to her chest as she communicates her process of tapping into her emotions. 'How does it feel to be part of a collective that holds us in our imperfections?' she repeats my question back to herself, reframing it as she does so. 'I'd say, how does it feel to have a friend that loves you? It's so transformative. We always say that it's the most valuable thing we have and that which we want to protect at all costs. Bare Minimum is often the only place any of us can show up in a vulnerable, messy way, and we don't take it for granted.'

The Bare Minimum Collective have offered immeasurable inspiration for Peaks of Colour. Their manifesto has guided our practice to ensure we don't just deliver rest for our communities but model it too. Our own set of evolving principles, for example, serve as a helpful reminder for the days when we feel somewhat astray in our work. They allow us to ground ourselves in a self-defined state of being and return to that place when external circumstances cause us to feel unmoored. This was an uncomfortable deconditioning at first, but slowing down to a steady pace is becoming easier, with less self-admonishing. Now we step trustingly through the portal of possibility, with faith that we will emerge with a greater capacity for creative imagination and future-building upon our return.

Our desire to simply rest in nature as a remedy for racial and gendered trauma catapulted us into the Right to Roam movement, which advocates that access to open space and reconnection with the natural world should be a right for all. We quickly realised that racial, gendered and land justice are intrinsically linked. We can't obtain one without the other, and it's for this reason that we included 'Nature-Led Practice' as one of our core principles, centring the intuition that arises when being of and with the land. It means we embrace the playful silliness, the awe, wonder and joy that can be found in nature and infuse our abolitionist practice with these lessons. The possibilities that arise when we listen to our exhaustion and follow natured ways of being often look like subtle, simple openings. This is what creates space for us to centre rest in our work. Making sure our meetings take place outside, either on a walk, or sat in a field — as much as the Sheffield weather will permit — is one such example.

Alternatively, these openings could be vast and porous, pushing us to delve into the intricacies and complexities of the natural world and completely transforming the ways we approach an issue or understand our role in the movement in the process. The introduction of 'seasonal organising' to our practice exemplifies this. Recognising that to survive the seasons you must change with them, Peaks of Colour mirrors the ways that nature has periods of emergence, abundance, rest and decay, operating on a seasonal structure that means we are not being productive 365 days of the year.

The summer months are when we bloom, offering walkshops series, collaborative events and spaces for reimagining healing in the Peaks. Come October, however, we go into hibernation and pause our external delivery to focus on organisational introspection and depth. In our first year of trialling this approach, seasonal organising looked like spending the autumn working on funding bids and developing our financial infrastructure – areas so out of my comfort zone that to do them alongside the activities of the summer would have been soul-crushing. In our second year, this looked like the intentional softness required of growing a new team. It is our hope that one day our 'hibernation' will be just that, uninterrupted pause, complete stillness, where we are able to do nothing but rest. In the meantime, we create space for the foundational building work and emerge again in spring with a renewed outlook, rested momentum and new series of walkshops to announce to the community.

I was humbled by how readily the community supported this decision, and now I cringe at how difficult it was to make initially. Heavily conditioned by working within a charity sector that normalises overextension and martyrdom, centring my own needs in this work felt uncomfortable and unnatural. I felt selfish and worried that the community would reject us, or that they'd have forgotten about us by the time we returned. This couldn't have been further from the truth. Each spring we re-emerge to a community that has anticipated our return and is excited for our next season of offerings, a community that supports the organisers' rest and is inspired also to approach their winters with a restful intention. What might happen if we were *all* to consider the ways we could take a seasonal approach to the work that matters to us most? What if we were to build resilient ecosystems that can sustain momentum even in periods of slowness? How might our bodies and brains and the work itself be transformed by periods of cyclical rest and retreat? Of emergence and re-engagement?

Yet for decades I worked through winters, sat on the edge of my bed in the blue hues of dawn, as in *Blue Monday*, expected to

maintain the same level of productivity while my brain disinte-
grated into the congealed slime that is seasonal depression. Our
bodies are seasonal vessels, and I ignored the signs. My mind and
body would scream at me to rest, disassociating and detaching
from the material realities of each day in the hope that I would
simply give in and return to my bed. But institutional pressure
would see me crawling to work, a daily act of harm.

Through a racial, gendered and land justice lens, our reimagin-
ation of *Blue Monday* would, with a wave of a magic wand,
transport our subject to the bank of her river, her arms supporting her as she dips a tentative toe into the icy stream. Blue, once
the colour of oppression, becomes transformed into the colour of
liberation. Tranquil, unpolluted waters reflecting the beaming sky.
Clouds dance above her head, while a carpet of nodding bluebells
sway gently in the meadow around her. Behind, hills surround
her. Blue tits can be heard from the neighbouring oak tree and
dragonflies flutter their emerald wings past blinking eyelashes.
Paul Robeson, Hattie McDaniel, Breonna Taylor, and every other
Black and person of colour reduced to the stereotype of their suffering would join her too. And, though the river may just keep
rolling along, it carries with it our blues and transforms them into
iridescent portals of possibility under the midday sun.

Rest as Resistance

Another organisation that has been influential in transforming
our understanding of rest is The Nap Ministry. Founded in 2016
by Tricia Hersey, this expansive organisation examines the liberatory power of naps through Collective Napping Experiences. Their
work utilises performance art, immersive workshops, site-specific
installations and community organising to instil safe spaces for
collective rest. Speaking in an online seminar on the importance

of visual representations of rest, Tricia references photographic portraits that depict her draped in lemon-yellow robes, dozing on a four-poster bed amid fields of cotton. 'Part of our art practice and part of our liberation practice is also aesthetic and uplifting the idea of seeing Black bodies, marginalised bodies, at rest,' she begins. 'This is a radical thought in an America, in a Western world that's anti-Black, where racism is rampant, where white supremacy is part of our making.'[22]

In her book *Rest as Resistance*, Hersey unpacks this further. Describing Black bodies as a commodified resource exploited as America's first experiment into how far they could push humans, she explores the ways that 'grind culture', as we know it today, is nothing more than a continuation of the white supremacy and capitalism that was established during slavery. 'When you don't see a lot of life (rest), death (grinding) becomes the alternative.'[23]

Alongside the already detrimental health consequences of exhaustion, Hersey argues that we also experience what she calls 'DreamSpace theft'. 'Daydreaming is not lazy, but an opportunity to heal, reset, grieve and imagine [...] there has been no space for any of us to dream of anything outside of what we have been born into,' Tricia writes. 'There is a massive knowledge and wisdom lying dormant in our exhausted and weary bodies and hearts [...] It is a time to be free from the confines of linear and grounded reality. To rest in a DreamSpace,'[24] she continues, 'is a red brick through the glass window of capitalism [and] dreaming becomes the prescription and balm needed to sustain this rest resistance long term.'[25]

In centring daydreaming as a collective form of rest, The Nap Ministry offers Collective Napping Experiences, which transform spaces – from yoga studios to art galleries, public parks to churches – into communal havens. These spaces are evidence that rest can be experienced anywhere. Those who attend these napping experiences can expect to be engulfed within rooms adorned with yoga mats, pillows, blankets and candles around an altar containing fresh flowers, cotton branches and archival photos of Black people. Then with music, affirmations, ritual and soundscapes, Tricia directs people into a state in which they feel safe to give in to sleep.

These Collective Napping Experiences give people the permission to be vulnerable, to pause, to centre self-care and to let someone else hold you. What emerges from these spaces, Tricia writes, is raw emotion.

She describes the physical release people feel after engaging with the parts of themselves they encounter while in deep rest, how this awakening reduces them to tears and how unaware they were of the intensity of their exhaustion until given a shame-free, guilt-free space to nap. This moment of pause, she writes, offers so much insight.

Despite being able to understand the deeply political theory of rest, and the embodied yearning of an exhausted body for restorative sleep, napping remains something that doesn't come naturally to me. Just as my bedtime routine is regularly peppered with restless flashbacks and intrusive thoughts, so are my attempts to nap. A particular set of circumstances is needed for me to nod off in the day: complete darkness – or the warmth of direct sunlight glaring on my face, a sofa with blankets, a teddy to cuddle and voices on the TV talking in the distance. Even then, I always struggle with completing a sleep cycle. Setting an alarm offers immediate time pressure, and I find myself staring at the ceiling, acutely aware of how awake I am. Or, if I don't set an alarm and manage to doze off, I'll invariably wake up outside my sleep cycle and jolt upright into an immediate panic attack that lingers for the rest of the day.

And so it was with a mixture of envy, awe and admiration that I was drawn to Simin, a community organiser I met during a weekend retreat for activists of colour, hosted by Decolonising Economics. Nestled in the Derbyshire hills, the weekend was designed to be a space where organisers of colour could escape for connection and rejuvenation. During our first day we cuddled up on sofas and perched cross-legged on cushions with soon-to-be friends, while the Decolonising Economics duo Guppi and Noni prompted us to take turns introducing ourselves in ways that didn't centre our work or activism. Sim introduced herself, and her pronouns. 'Annnnnnnddddddd . . .' she paused, nodding assuredly into her lap before the words tumbled out of her. 'And for the past couple of months I've been taking twelve-hour naps – well, trying to, at least. It's kind of an experiment I'm having with myself. I'm enjoying it!' She beamed at the room, shoulders dropping with release, as if she'd just shared a secret that she'd been holding back for some time.

A couple of months later, we sat opposite each other again, on screen this time. When Sim speaks, she does so with considered and measured intention, pausing intermittently before conveying words of purpose. With every syllable, I feel as if I am witnessing the kind of vulnerability in which ego knows no place and am invited into a raw understanding of who Sim is. She tells me of her difficulty identifying and naming her experiences of burnout, and how she only became conscious of it when her partner observed and named it for her. Sim is a personal assistant for chronically ill and disabled queer people who live locally to her and a member of Radical Routes, a network of housing co-ops across the country. Like many of us in activist and organising spaces, she wears multiple hats and juggles varied roles in an attempt to find a balance between passion and income.

A common thread that runs through all Sim's roles is care. Her work is heavy with physical and emotional labour, and we talked about the ways that the professionalisation of care positions it as a transactional commodity rather than something reciprocal and mutual. When you're the person constantly giving care and seldom receiving it back, exhaustion feels like an inevitability. The impact of this, Sim tells me, is that she often struggles to juggle her own responsibilities, feel grounded in her relationships or meet her own care needs. Earlier that year, however, two situations ignited a new commitment to developing a better understanding of herself and her body's need for rest.

The first was when her housemate caught Covid and Sim was required to stay home and isolate with them, and it was then that she realised how burnt out she was. 'When my housemate started testing negative and we were able to come out of quarantine, I didn't really want to leave! I was still really happy with staying in my bedroom,' she tells me, 'having a bit of a routine, but otherwise doing very little, just being in my own space. I found that I really thrived in it. Even with my reluctance to name it as burnout, the way my mind and body embraced rest probably says it all.' She sent a text message to her then-boss describing her experiences, then took a prolonged period off work. 'That is where the twelve-hour nap started,' she tells me. 'It felt really scary at the time to think beyond my current existence, that kind of safe place that I'd built for myself at home, and I found myself worrying about whether I could ever go back to work now that this has been real-ised. But taking some time off allowed me to push that to the back of my mind for a few months at least. I just started . . . napping! I wouldn't set an alarm. I'd let my body wake up when it wanted to and if I still felt sleepy, I'd maybe go to the toilet, have a bite to eat and go back to napping.'

I ask her what benefits she's noticed in herself as a result of the experiment and she beams, the list leaping out of her before I can even finish my sentence. 'The difference looks like being in my body more, feeling like I can choose to support the things that I want to do, and I can choose not to support the things that I don't want to. I'm better at saying "no" to stuff. Sometimes I turned down jobs to prioritise ones that relieve significant financial pressure and create space for rest. And now I just think, "Whoah, with that amount of money, I can now do all the other things I want to do. I can sleep when I want to!" I don't have this giant sinking feeling in my stomach where it just feels like so much stress.' She motions slow circles around her stomach. 'My gastrointestinal digestion often affects how I can eat or how hungry I feel, but I don't feel like my body's in flames any more. Yeah. I feel more relaxed, more at ease.'

'What it's given me is agency,' she explains, 'and I think the more I learn about myself in relation to my autism, the more I understand how important agency is.' This was the second situation which offered Sim a new lens to understand rest. 'One of the traits of autism that I came across last year is called PDA. It stands for pathological demand avoidance – whatever that means – but I like to reframe it as "Persistent Drive for Autonomy".' Dismissing problematic medical terminology with a wave of her hand, Sim explains that traditionally this label is placed on autistic children who struggle to meet the demands placed on them, such as brushing their teeth or going to bed at a certain time. For adults, these demands are multiple and varied, from putting the wash on, to paying your taxes, eating three balanced meals a day or meeting social expectations.

'Reframing it as a need for autonomy feels good to me. I struggle with "productivity culture" because that inherently forces me to put a demand on myself that I can't meet, and then I get paralysed and stuck. In the end, I might only achieve one thing. But actually, when I've got autonomy, I'm going to do ten other things all while meeting my own basic needs, stretching my body, going outside, gardening and fitting in a nap.' On how she's found maintaining a culture of napping since returning to work, Sim smiles, 'Now I do it as much as I can manage realistically around my schedule, but somehow, since I've come back to work, I've managed to make it sustainable. I now nap with my partner, for example, and working on a freelance schedule definitely helps. This isn't like an exact twelve-hour thing, sometimes it can be eight hours, sometimes it could be like fourteen, fifteen. I try not to keep track too much, but I'd say on average I still manage to get twelve. I hadn't thought about it too much, but somehow napping has just become a priority for me now.'

Sim's napping revelations, The Bare Minimum's approach to work and organising, Tricia Hersey's pioneering of rest and Peaks of Colour's centring of nature connectedness may feel unruly, unrealistic, or unattainable to many of us. Yet through a lens of autonomy, the way these individuals and collectives prioritise personal and collective needs exemplifies how exhaustion is not something our bodies and minds would choose for us. In elevating our understanding of activist burnout, we amplify the severity of the condition, recognising how it is intentionally weaponised to create conditions in which we exist in a living death. To extend ourselves the permission to carve out space and time for a rest is a defiant act that rejects fatigue as an inherited inevitability. This is how we can redefine napping, pausing, slowing and dreaming as things that are not lazy or passive, but conscious and active. Much like the transformative power of the blues, rest offers a way to transcend our exhaustion into radical possibilities, something capitalism would much rather we confine only to the corners of our imagination.

Case Study #1: The Home

It is no accident that this homeplace, as fragile and
as transitional as it may be, a makeshift shed, a
small bit of earth where one rests, is always subject
to violation and destruction. For when a people no
longer have the space to construct homeplace, we
cannot build a meaningful community of resistance
— bell hooks[1]

Maslow's Hierarchy of Needs is a tool created by psychologist Abraham Maslow, which identifies the basic and advanced needs that must be actualised for people to live a sustainable, dignifying, affirming life. The home can be understood as an institution that transcends all five of the needs in Maslow's Hierarchy: a place of shelter and reproduction (physiological); property and personal security (safety); family and sense of connection (love and belonging); and freedom and self-worth (esteem), all of which nurture us to become the truest, most fulfilled versions of ourselves (self-actualisation).

That the home functions in the best interests of those who inhabit it is, therefore, an integral requirement for a burnout-free existence. For when the home fails to do so, it can present a site of structural and material deprivation, adverse socialisation, interpersonal violence and ecological unsafety. Amid the post-pandemic landscape, the cost-of-living crisis and multiple other socio-political crises, however, the home's foundational ability to nurture and nourish is crumbling from numerous directions and it is becoming increasingly hard for us to rely on it to meet our basic needs. It's for this reason that, in our exploration of how burnout is a pervasive issue facilitated by institutional violence, the home is the first case study we delve into here. These deep dives punctuate our emotional explorations, in order to validate the feelings we experience under racial capitalism and remind us that it is society, and not us, that is defective. They can be read as complementary to the emotional chapters, or alone.

Home as a Refuge
In the UK:

- 1 in 3 women have experienced domestic abuse;
- 1 in 3 people who have been raped have experienced it in their own home;
- 1 in 7 children experience abuse at the hands of a family member.

Being both a domestic abuse survivor and a practitioner within the VAWG sector, gendered violence is the first thing that comes to mind when I consider the home as a potential site of burnout. In her book *A Feminist Theory of Violence*, French political scientist Françoise Vergès offers a decolonial perspective on gendered violence. Vergès examines gendered violence at its source, which includes racial capitalism, populism, imperialism and the proliferation of prisons. Violence, she explains, has a structural element in which the dynamics of power and control that a perpetrator plays upon are reinforced by a wider culture of violence.

The government's dismissal during lockdown of abuse as a private issue, rather than one of public responsibility, is just one example of this in action. As we were confined to our homes as a place of 'sanctuary' amid the dangers of the outside world, the National Domestic Abuse Helpline witnessed a 65 per cent increase in calls within the first few months of the pandemic. This amplifies the truths that survivors know too well: the home can become a place of hurt rather than healing, of isolation rather than community, of a diminishing of self rather than self-actualisation. So much of the language around survivorship centres around seeking refuge – a place providing safety or shelter from danger and harm. It makes being denied refuge in the place we're told is inherently safe even more sinister.

Towards the end of my career in the VAWG sector, I specialised in the intersections of racial and gendered violence experienced by LGBTQ+ people of colour. As survivors within this demographic, our experiences of domestic abuse are compounded by our race, culture, gender and sexual identity. We're also more likely to experience violence from multiple networks – our partners, families, friends, wider communities, the state – and are less likely to receive culturally competent support from services, meaning the risk of institutional harm is disproportionately greater. It's a system dominated by carceral feminist politics, a type of (often white, liberal, mainstream) feminism that is oppositional to abolitionism due to its advocacy for the expansion of prisons and sentencing in response to issues such as gendered violence. In this system only 2 per cent of rape cases see their perpetrators charged, let alone convicted, underlining how the so-called 'healing' and 'justice' afforded to our white, cis, heterosexual counterparts represents a woefully inadequate and unattainable outcome for us.

Vergès reminds us that 'the recent mobilisation against gender-based and sexual violence offers a theoretical and practical opportunity: that of making this violence the very terrain on which to challenge patriarchal capitalism'.[2] What might it look like, for example, if we were to examine harms within the home not only through the more overt lenses of domestic abuse and sexual violence, but via the more subtle and multifaceted ways that structural violence is concentrated and repurposed within its walls?

Home as a Microcosm

By understanding the home in this way, as a microcosm that encapsulates the characteristics of society at large, we can see how it is impossible to explore anything relating to burnout without looking at the normative family structures and gender roles within the home. 'The idea of a perfect home is one which opposes any autonomy or flexibility or deviation from a normative expression of identity – all the things that are intrinsic to queerness. It's this "perfect home" construct that denied me a truly supportive support system,' Jasmine Isa Qureshi tells me. Jasmine is a writer, researcher, marine biologist and founder of Soil to Sky, an organisation that centres intersectional Queer Ecologies in its work.

Over Zoom, we discuss how the home is defined by patriarchy as a space of care, which a traditional, nuclear family is said to uphold. Care becomes a feminine quality through the assumption of gender binaries which value cis-heteronormativity and devalue gender-expansive or non-conforming identities. Through its intersection with racism, classism, homophobia, transphobia, ableism and ageism, patriarchy delegates roles, power and status in a way that ultimately oppresses us all, but particularly women and queer people of colour.[5] 'We're brought up to believe that the systems we live in are binary, but Queer Ecology unveils how non-binary nature can be. It's the unlearning of systemic biases and embracing a diversity of thought and experience,' Jasmine says.

In the 1980s, sociologist Arlie Hochschild, whose work explores the 'sociology of emotion', introduced us to the ways normative family structures reinforce gender roles, which then produce an unequal division of labour. Hochschild found that while men were only expected to contribute to paid work, women, comparatively, were responsible for a 'second shift'. Upon returning from paid labour as part of a capitalist workforce, they were also expected to do unpaid housework and childcare, shouldering the responsibility for practical and emotional labour. A recent UN report documenting the progress of the 'Sustainable Development Goals' captured how, globally, women continue to spend an average of 2.8 more hours a day than men on unpaid care and domestic work.[4] However, amid abject state-abandonment in the UK, where rising childcare costs and working from home blurs the lines in a work–life balance, the figures rise to an average of 4 hours a day, 60 per cent more unpaid work than men.[5]

Hochschild reflected on how this burden of care has been an unintended consequence of a second-wave feminism that was preoccupied with achieving women's equal access and participation in a male-dominated capitalist system. Alternatively, an intersectional approach that strives for liberation, as opposed to equality, urges us to imagine beyond the limitations of this white feminist aspiration. Black Feminist Patricia Hill Collins, for instance, suggests that 'just as the traditional family ideal provides a rich site for understanding intersectional inequalities, reclaiming alternative family structures may provide an intriguing and important site of resistance.'[6]

Reflecting on how, as queer people, we build our own communities of care, particularly when biological families fail, Jasmine offers chosen families in queer communities as an example of how this resistance manifests. 'Chosen families are not new, they have been modelled by indigenous communities for centuries. But when colonial forces saw how powerful this was, they set about dismantling indigenous structures as a means of control, of removing autonomy and building a hierarchy,' she explains. 'Chosen families are a resistance to this, they're the dissolution of capitalism, and of this efficiency-based model, in favour of an ecosystem of care. This is key to mutual aid and community.'

Home as (In)Justice

Like so many of our efforts to resist the capitalist status quo, however, when we forge homes on our own terms, the dominant system will often find ways to repress it. 'It's almost like a supportive home is a reward for conformity,' Jasmine continues, 'and anyone who doesn't – queer people, single parents, childless families – are penalised, socially and relationally. We're told only certain people are allowed to have a home and burnout is the punishment.' Abolitionist collective Cradle agrees: 'If you are living with people who're not related to you, the landlord's got to apply for a specific kind of licence [House in Multiple Occupation], so nuclear families and straight people are usually favoured,' they write.[7] In *Brick by Brick: How We Build a World Without Prisons*, they detail how housing injustice, i.e. the material deprivation of insecure and unsafe housing, presents a health and social justice issue. Yet, despite capitalism positioning home ownership as evidence of productivity, housing insecurity within the UK is rampant. While wages have stagnated, over the past twenty years housing prices have tripled. Meanwhile, skyrocketing utility bills have doubled throughout the cost-of-living crisis, and in the past year alone the cost of rent has increased by up to 15 per cent.[8] As a result, working people are closer to homelessness than home ownership, with Shelter reporting that throughout 2023, homelessness rose by 14 per cent.

Even when we are housed, the safety, security and stability of a home's material brick and mortar cannot be guaranteed within our current political climate. Housing campaigner Kwajo Tweneboa uses social media to expose the damp, mouldy, polluted, rotting and rodent-infested conditions that are commonplace in rented properties across the UK. The realities captured by Tweneboa's ongoing documentation seldom make the headlines. When they do, it's likely as a result of abject tragedy and suffering. The Grenfell Tower fire – where in 2017 seventy-two people were killed when a fire broke out in a twenty-four-storey block of flats in North Kensington – is a haunting example of this. The blaze, which lasted three days, was started by an electrical fault, then accelerated by dangerously combustible aluminium composite cladding. A public inquiry found that the tower block – whose residents were disproportionately people of colour – was unsafe, and that a number of residents had complained to the council months earlier, highlighting the fire risk the building posed.

Rather than address the chronic housing crisis and remedy this issue, the government reinforces othering and alienation, through, for example, the gentrification of working-class neighbourhoods and the privatisation of social housing. Cradle recounts the multiple ways housing insecurity is used to police and punish marginalised communities. This ranges from how Gypsy, Roma and Travellers are being forced into homelessness through the new Police, Crime, Sentencing and Courts Act, to the ways entire families were forcibly evicted from social housing as punishment for young people's participation in the 2021 London riots. They point to Margaret Thatcher's Right to Buy scheme in the 1980s, which allowed tenants to purchase their council homes, as influencing the increasingly punitive housing policies we see today. As a result, the government's concern lies predominantly in private property ownership rather than providing affordable public housing.

'These conditions on static residence do not derive from nature but rather from capitalist notions of property and "hard work" [...] While asset ownership has been sold to our generation as a substitute safety net, the privatisation of social housing and rising housing prices have made this unattainable for the vast majority,' they write.[9] The consequences of such policies extend far beyond the physical house itself; a stable address is required when accessing healthcare, obtaining a passport, finding a job, or being granted parole in prison, which means our ability to possess secure, safe shelter also impacts our ability to access other life-affirming services. When the roofs over our heads are used as a political bargaining chip that fuels greed, competition and scarcity, is it any wonder we burn out?

Home as an Ecology

Amid so many systemic failures preoccupied with ownership for the few, Cradle remind us that at the heart of abolitionist praxis is the stewarding of safe landscapes in which we can all belong. This means ensuring our homes, neighbourhoods and wider environments are built through infrastructures of care. In our consideration of what it means to reside in a space free from burnout, this Venn diagram of factors helps us see how land and environmental justice become integral to our understanding of home. It's here we are introduced to the meaning of 'ecology'. Defined as the study of relationships among living organisms, including humans and their physical environment, 'ecology' comes from the Latin and Greek origins of 'eco', meaning 'home' or 'household'. An ecological consideration, therefore, broadens our understanding of home beyond buildings or the connections which reside within them, to include the reciprocal relationship with the wider environment we inhabit.

In recent years, there has been no shortage of cases evidencing the dangers of a mutually destructive relationship with our environment. One unforgettable example is Ella Kissi-Debrah from Lewisham, who died in 2013, aged nine, as a result of acute respiratory failure, severe asthma and – as a coroner who made legal history seven years later ruled – air pollution exposure, with traffic emissions identified as the principal source. Ella was exposed to levels of nitrogen dioxide that exceeded both the EU and UK's legal limits, and particulate matter pollution that exceeded the guidance offered by the World Health Organization.

We can understand Ella's death as a consequence of environmental racism – where intersecting environmental and socio-economic inequalities disproportionately impact racialised communities. It also signifies the emerging health and environmental crises that are occurring as a consequence of centuries of refusing to consider our environment as home, and our more-than-human kin as family. The ways neoliberal, patriarchal, racial capitalism sever a connection that might otherwise be used to foster both emotional and ecological repair means that the solution to this problem cannot possibly be found through such prisms. Frameworks such as Queer Ecology, however, allow those of us who have been excluded from our natural homes the opportunity to redefine our connections with them.

'Queer Ecology is a perspective, a way of perceiving and understanding ecology, and thus, a different way of perceiving existence. Because ecology then links to biology, biology then links to the systemic biases that people have come up with over time to govern and rule – like gender binaries, racial hierarchies and other such nonsense,' Jasmine explains. 'Our biggest example is how a Western science has prescribed gender norms to nature. But the clownfish, for example, dispute this because they change sex when the numbers of inseminators or the numbers of egg layers in the group rise and fall. From that we learn that nature doesn't view gender identifiers or markers as set in stone, nor does it apply gender norms or gender roles to the organisms with those identifiers.'

Jasmine and I get distracted from the questions I have before me, and we muse over how our perception of the natural world often mirrors our view of the homes in which we reside. I reflect upon how fitting it is that Sheffield, also known as the Green City due to its proximity to nature, should be the place I found refuge after fleeing an abusive relationship, and she tells me that as a trans, Muslim, Indian, Pakistani, non-binary woman who hasn't seen or spoken to her family in a long time, she too finds nature to be her surrogate home.

'This is why access to natural spaces is such an amazing thing. An ecosystem is non-judgemental, so it's easy to feel at home when in nature. I think this is why the powers that be have facilitated such a disconnect with it,' Jasmine considers. 'This brings us back to this idea of community. Nature, its environmental biodiversity and ecosystems are the best example of community. Within an ecosystem every part has to be content – otherwise you risk ecosystem unbalance. Ecosystems teach us reciprocity, symbiosis.

What we can observably learn from nature is this idea that home is a community where everyone is content, and everything has autonomy while being responsible to and for each other.'

Returning to nature teaches us how it feels to belong in our bodies, with each other and the earth. This autonomy, Jasmine says, permits comfort, and it's where we can comfortably be ourselves that comes to feel like home. By centring the lived experiences of those most likely to burn out within the home, and exploring expansive avenues of thought such as Queer Ecology, the possibilities of our homemaking can become expansive. Creating ecologies of care is essential for revolutionary practice. After all, we cannot resist systems of oppression if we're being subjected to living conditions that are abusive, exploitative, unsafe and insecure. Ensuring that our basic needs are met, through safe and accessible housing for all, through healthy and affirming relationships, through care that is cultivated and shared on an egalitarian basis,[10] means that we can access rest and replenish ourselves in order to return to the fight. This is how we lay the foundations for a burnout-free society.

On Radical Grief

I'm aware that I and people I love may perish in the
morning, but there's a light on our faces now. And if you
live in the shadow of death, it gives you a certain freedom.
— James Baldwin[1]

Grief may seem like an unusual emotion to feature in our discussion of burnout, yet it might just be the most important. Grief, after all, is the one universal trauma. No matter our race, class, age, background, gender or sexuality, we will all find ourselves touched by it eventually. Grief, however, is held by the West in a robotic capacity. Nobody really knows what to do with you when you're grieving, and while people may extend a hand to pat you on the back tentatively, muttering uncomfortable *there-theres*, there is so often an unspoken desire for everyone to put up and shut up. We are expected to soldier on, persevering despite the crushing, breathless weight of loss. How could something so unnatural result in anything but burnout?

Even in employment law, there's no legal statutory guidance obliging employers to grant paid bereavement leave for personal losses. The average number of bereavement days you're likely able to receive ranges from three to fourteen, depending on your relative proximity to the deceased. Two weeks. Two weeks to get over the immediate and infinite absence of a parent, a partner, a best friend, a grandparent, a sibling. Two weeks is seldom enough time to process the shock, the sorrow, the pain, to alert family, to make funeral arrangements. Two weeks isn't enough space to have a series of firsts without that person, experience a good day shielded by moments of forgetting, followed by sleepless nights of relentless remembering. Two weeks doesn't account for the hours spent combing through photo albums and wiping soft tears off the images. The inevitable falling out and making up with family members. The laughing, the crying, choosing flower arrangements and being thrust into the overwhelming world of legalities, wills, finances. And for the losses that don't fit the traditional mould – a miscarriage, a friendship or relationship breakdown; the loss of yet another piece of the natural world; a woman walking home late at night taken by the hands of violent men; for our trans siblings, for whom, as Alok V. Menon describes, 'every day I walk outside is a leap outside of faith. Sometimes I wonder if I'll be the next statistic';[2] or entire communities made disposable to war and world politics – there is nothing.

Capitalism doesn't know how to accommodate such a raw and violent emotion. *Cope quickly*, it tells us. *Your grief is an inconvenience, so return to work with enough cognitive dissonance that you don't disrupt the functionality of your place of employment.* We must bury the grief, to ensure it doesn't overspill and touch the person next to us, whose grief is also buried and must not be disturbed. Otherwise, what may occur is a domino effect where the dormant grief erupts out of each of us. An awakening to all that we had suppressed and forgotten. A contagion that unlocks the deepest sorrows within us and spreads. An epidemic of mourning. A national crisis.

The Covid-19 pandemic is a poignant example of this. We all lost something during this time: our loved ones, our freedom, the illusion of immortality, the frivolities that allowed us to feel like life had meaning, or the comfortable façade that for decades has told us that we, the West, were superior, untouchable, invincible. It's a grief that will likely have consequences for generations to come, yet we have not even begun to quantify, measure or address the scale and impact of it. We were urged by bumbling politicians to 'return to normal' as a patriotic duty, yet the ability to package grief into an individualistic box is a privilege rarely afforded to communities of colour. Too often our personal heartbreak is entwined with the political enforcement of a harmful existence. We become voyeurs of our own grief: we watch people who look like us beg for breath then die at the hands of police brutality in real time on national TV, see our loved ones perish under subpar Covid regulations, witness institutional violence ravish our communities, and watch as our homes disintegrate due to the lack of environmental protections. All while those elsewhere, the privileged, the un-persecuted, observe with pity, and think, *I'm glad that's not me.*

We know too that our unresolved grief has socio-political consequences. In the UK, for example, 91 per cent of adult men in prisons have experienced six or more losses, with traumatic bereavements (such as those caused by murder or suicide) experienced by more than three-quarters of incarcerated males.[3] Loved ones, deceased. Former selves, changed. Communities, fractured. Homelands, displaced. Histories, destroyed. Our grief is intergenerational, woven into the fabric of our DNA, suspended in mid-air, just out of our reach, to be examined, discussed, then moulded into something palatable to an online audience of white guilt.

There's a sinister subtlety to how our traumas as people of colour are routinely mined and repackaged as 'opportunities'. Yet the ways this unfolded in the weeks and months that followed George Floyd's murder were obnoxiously loud. Overnight, our lived experiences were platformed and our self-professed allies flocked like vultures: black squares on Instagram feeds, colourful infographics spouting James Baldwin quotes, endless Q&As, poorly paid think-pieces, equality, diversity and inclusion (EDI) trainings, and book clubs. Eventually, inevitably, people became desensitised to our grief. Anti-racism became boring, the reality of abolition was too much of a responsibility and our allies ran for the hills, guilt assuaged. Contrastingly, Black communities emerged personally, politically and professionally scarred, and, when the dust settled, we were able to see just how little meaningful change was made during this time.

As activists the grief we carry will often inform our direction and approach to movement-building. When we enter this work either as a flame, raw in our vulnerabilities, or singed around the edges, we're already halfway to burnout. If not cared for, the pain we carry has the potential to be transformed into harmful practice, rather than regenerative change. Describing grief as the necessary ingredient of a revolutionary imagination, writer and sociologist Gargi Bhattacharyya reminds us that without grief, though held collectively, we cannot remain open to our profound interdependence. 'Address grief as a personal wound, something to make us stronger, an opportunity to display that most dubious of attributes, resilience, and the tiny cracks through which collective redemption might seep begin to close up,' she writes.[4]

My own exploration of grief work as an extension of my burnout recovery is still in its infancy. I find myself tiptoeing around the edges, observing with intrigue and sampling the array of possible outlets, hopeful that one, or more, sticks. What has become clear, however, is that forging spaces for collective grief feels like a pressing responsibility – to ourselves and to each other. But how do we build spaces and structures that permit us the time and space to hold, process, navigate and heal from our grief as a community?

During their first in-person panel event since lockdown, Healing Justice London convened with the brilliance behind MAIA, Civic Square, RESOLVE and Kin Structures – all groups whose community work, rooted in arts and culture, is in service of building and sustaining life-affirming infrastructures at scale. Together, they explored how we might build different kinds of infrastructures that are 'conducive to life, dignity, safety and joy'. As the panellists demonstrated alternative models, methodologies and practices that brought seemingly abstract dreams to material reality, what struck me was the implication that within a society where our life is affirmed, so too are our experiences of and interactions with death.

During the event, the founder of MAIA, Amahra Spence, described societal ills as collective cracks, in an echo of Bhattacharyya. 'We need more breaks, more cracks, more tears,' she said, urging us to see these crevices as opportunities. 'We need to get so much more comfortable and brave about being uncomfortable. Our wounds have been portals for all of us. Our wounds have birthed capoeira, hip-hop, dumplings! How do we tend to those wounds?'[5] Grief, and the ways we are unsupported to learn from it, sit with it, move with it, heal from it, is a wound which has been festering on the white skin of the British Isles for centuries. I find myself tantalisingly fascinated in how we can suture it. How can we build a bridge over the canyon, plant seeds in the cracks, create a thing of beauty from what is broken?

Grief as Kintsugi

When I was a child I had a somewhat creepy obsession with collecting porcelain dolls. Adorned in lace and bows, these ornate figurines, with coiffed ringlets and intricately woven dresses, transformed my bedroom into something out of a scene from a horror movie. The day I outgrew them was the day that I threw each doll around my bedroom in a fit of misplaced rage. Afterwards, my mum and I swept the broken fragments of their rosy-cheeked faces into the bin, and I remember feeling guilty and ashamed. But mostly, I felt self-pity. For in each broken porcelain face I saw myself. Not yet a teenager, yet equally broken beyond repair.

In Japan, there is a practice called *kintsugi*, whereby broken pottery isn't seen as disposable or a write-off, but is instead mended using melted gold to bind the pieces back together. Because it's the emotion I recognise I'm the most disconnected from, I've become attuned to my desire to reach a healthy relationship with the cracks of my grief. Compelling in its imperfections, beautiful in its repair, this patchworked crockery is how I would like my relationship with grief to feel.

As a child I could never comprehend death, and for the most part I still don't. Nowadays I generally straddle indifference and disassociation, rather than acceptance. Despite attending a secular primary school that prided itself on its multiculturalism and multi-faith teaching, stories of Jesus were as frequent as the seasons. Images of him dying on the cross would send me into spirals of overthinking and over-empathising. I couldn't comprehend how a person could go from living to being nothing. Heaven, hell or any kind of imagined afterlife seemed too hypothetically indefinite to the little atheist that I was, and I couldn't make peace with the weirdly grotesque afterlife rituals either. *What do you mean you're going to lob someone you love into a hole or set them on fire?*

So when my estranged dad died, his death was beyond my eight-year-old reasoning. My mum wouldn't tell me how he died or let us attend his funeral. I assumed that this was due to some huge morbid secret, and I spent sleepless nights conjuring new and rare diseases in my imagination that would account for such secrecy. It turns out that the reason she hadn't told me was simply because she didn't know – his body was so decomposed when he was found that the coroner was unable to identify a cause of death. The only reason he was found at all is because neighbours began to identify a smell, not because he had family present enough to notice his absence – the violence he perpetrated against my mum ensured his isolation. She rightly assessed that this information would be too traumatising for a child, but after much pressure from me, she relented.

The day I had to run up the street to my grandparents' house to tell them that dad was in the garden pulling my mum's hair out was the last time I saw him. I was five. This is my only real memory of him, a memory I associate with the soundtrack of *Singing in the Rain*, the film I watched in the living room while the adults, and the police, sorted things out. Despite witnessing the abuse, I was many years away from an understanding of protection (otherwise known as restraining) orders and why I wasn't to see him again. So when he died, I felt bereft. And in many ways, I still do – not for the father-shaped gap he left behind, but certainly bereft of the sense of identity and ancestral connection to which he could have introduced me, and of the opportunity to not have my first relationship with a man be one of fear and distrust.

My dad was cremated, and from a town called Bridlington, we scattered his ashes in the sea. It was a ceremony my mum had hoped would bring closure but instead inspired me to draw scenes of a Black man lynched, tied to a bonfire like a witch being set on fire or laid at the bottom of the sea surrounded by fish. I couldn't understand death and for years I hated returning to the coast, afraid my dad would emerge from the ocean and start pulling out my mum's hair on the beach.

Not long after this my maternal grandfather, the only father figure I'd known, also died. He walked me and my little brother to the bus stop one Wednesday morning, and by the time the school bell rang at three o'clock he had taken his own life. I was twelve. My mum says I had always been an emotional child – 'just like me', she'd say. Predisposed, perhaps. Yet on that Wednesday, I found myself definitively catapulted out of childhood innocence and into the adult understanding that life is painful, so painful. I was consumed by this pain, and the pain of others: the pain my dad inflicted and the pain that somehow none of us realised my grandad was carrying.

With his death, any hope of having a stable foundation on which to build a healthy relationship with grief was annihilated. It not only introduced me to heartbreak, but also to the realisation that perhaps I didn't have to live with the pain. I went from a child who had never heard of suicide to suddenly being presented with the option of relieving my suffering, by way of taking my own life. A generational curse, enacted. Despite my mum doing every-thing to keep my grandad's death private, the *Doncaster Free Press* reported it. This was then seen by a girl in my class, a bullyish weasel of a child who took it upon herself to tell the entirety of the school bus in a relayed chain of whispers. Eventually someone – I can't quite remember who – gently told me the rumour that was circulating.

The details of that school journey remain a blur, overshadowed by the truth-revealing conversation I had with my mum when I got home later that day. My grandfather didn't leave a suicide note, so we were all left unable to make sense of the ways our perception of and relationship with him differed from his internal struggle. Regardless of how fluent I may now be in the complexities of trauma and mental health, I fear there will always be within me a little child who can't reconcile the jovial, silly, perpetually joking, seemingly carefree relationship I had with my grandad with the person who felt it necessary to take his own life on a Wednesday afternoon. With 'whys' that will never be answered, I find myself questioning whether I'll ever be able to reach a point of acceptance. Perpetually stuck between a state of bargaining and denial, at far too young an age I was catapulted into knowing that neither life nor death are particularly affirming.

Twenty years later, I find myself in a similar place to that young girl who took out her grief on her porcelain dolls. Though I now possess much less destructive tools with which to express my emotions, like so many of us I'm still trying to piece together the fragmented shrapnel of my relationship with grief, including the more recent loss of my grandma.

My granny and I shared the same name, an obsessive love of cats, ITV murder dramas and old Hollywood musicals. Following a gradual erasure of all her memories save for me, my mum and my brother, my grandma died in the April of 2020, as a result of complications associated with the deterioration of her dementia. Coinciding with the intense early days of the Covid crisis, our personal loss felt insignificant among the nation's collective grief, yet simultaneously all-consuming in a way which completely distorted the reality of the outside world. After my grandma died, I didn't speak for five days, my silence breaking only to express the 'anger' stage of grief at distant relatives.

Yet, it's not just a parent or grandparent that I'm grieving, but a childhood sheltered by youthful innocence, naïvety and wonder that I could have enjoyed had it not been for loss, and the versions of myself in adulthood I could have become had it not been for decades of gendered violence and racialised trauma.

I understand a big part of the healing and recovery ahead must be self-acceptance. Finding ways to restore the porcelain doll of my former childhood self and apply the unwavering belief that even though some damage may take a lifetime to repair (or is, perhaps, irreversible), it is possible for all of us to make something beautiful out of the brokenness.

For three decades my relationship with grief was one of spiritual and psychological avoidance. Perpetually in flight mode, I ensured I was severed from myself, my lost loved ones and my surroundings by running away – through the more socially acceptable mode of going backpacking the moment I turned eighteen. With the civil service pension I'd inherited from my dad (arguably the only good thing he ever did for me and my brother), I was able to actualise an escape that would have been inconceivable to me as a child of an extremely working-class, benefit-dependent, single-parent household. I would never have been able to attain the financial independence to travel otherwise. And travel I did. I interrailed across Europe, Iceland and North Africa. I backpacked through India, Sri Lanka and Nepal. I became skilled in compartmentalising the varied and multiple lives I was living, somehow able to complete an undergraduate and postgraduate degree while barely being in the country at all. Whether I was home or abroad, I was rarely present, sleepwalking through some of the most formative years, experiences, relationships, milestones of my life. I have very little recollection of any of it.

In many ways I resonate with the protagonist in Ottessa Moshfegh's *My Year of Rest and Relaxation*, an unnamed woman in her mid-twenties who embarks on a year-long sabbatical of rest. She bears little resemblance to me in terms of privilege and economic comfort, but her penchant for running away from her problems feels uncomfortably relatable. The character isn't a likeable one. On the surface she's selfish, bullying and narcissistic, using her inherited wealth and any relationship she encounters to achieve the luxury of time off. Her reasons for doing so could be interpreted as an attempt to reject the superficial, self-absorbed, unfulfilling life of a neoliberal millennial living in New York, for example. Yet while this protagonist isn't political enough to stage a resistance for collective good, *My Year of Rest and Relaxation* can also be interpreted as a commentary on grief's incompatibility with capitalism, on how we cannot grieve while interacting with it.

The main character is in the first stage of grief — denial — and is able to find a way of moving through the grief of losing both parents, with whom she shared a complicated relationship, without ever having to feel a thing. She tranquillises herself using a cocktail of prescription drugs prescribed by an unscrupulous psychiatrist. She isolates herself from her one friend, Reva, and the rest of the world. She ensures that any bridge associated with her old life, her career and colleagues burns. With dramatic anomie, she employs these self-destructive, reckless and manipulative methods to achieve the isolation that will allow her to mourn. This speaks to how few healthy avenues of grief are available to us under a capitalist system, and the lengths to which we must go to feel in control of our big feelings. Immature and callous as her approach may be, we can see it as a form of survival. This more generous interpretation of her motivations, then, view her determination to achieve sleep as symptomatic of a trauma response. 'My past life would be but a dream, and I could start over without regrets, bolstered by the bliss and serenity that would have accumulated in my year of rest and relaxation,' she writes.[6]

Arguably, the very same neoliberal structures that the protagonist is determined to flee from have caused us, in the West, to become so detached from our ability to grieve. Rather than allowing us to experience our grief as the intense, relational experience that it is, such systems of oppression minimise and individualise it. This hasn't always been the case. Though not without opportunity for ample critique, the periods of mourning observed in the Victorian period, for example, recognised loss as something which requires dedicated time. Mourners indicated their grief to those around them by wearing only black; the recommended duration of mourning was usually dependent on the closeness of the relationship and could be anything from six months to two years. Today, we find ourselves – through colonialism, imperialism and neoliberalism – segregated from ritual, from community, from emotion. And anyone who steps foot on British soil is also often expected to relinquish – or at the very least conceal – their grieving rituals and ceremonies in the name of assimilation.

When a 'normal' or 'healthy' relationship with grief (as normal or as healthy as a Western relationship with grief can be) feels lost to so many of us, looking to self-practices that sit outside of capitalism's parameters can help us to reconnect with our sadness and pain. On the collective grief we are sharing amid the ongoing suffering of multiple communities around the world, Tuvaluan psychotherapist Leah Manaema Avene reminds us of the generative indigenous solutions that can keep our bodies and communities safe and strong. 'My understanding of grief is that it is love with nowhere to go [...] so when I trace my grief to the love underneath, I can give that somewhere to go, I can go out in my community, I can care for people [...] Every time we have faith and every time we lean in for connection we are resisting this system.'[7] So many of us are disconnected from the memory of any indigenous or ancestral grief practice. There has been a generational series of forgetting.

Grief as Cracks in't Concrete

As children, cracks in the pavement were considered bad luck: '*If you stand on a crack, you break your back. If you stand on a line, you marry a swine,*' we'd chant melodically. We'd leap over these severed slabs of concrete, relieved that we were to live another day with spine and future love life intact. Yet if grief is to be our metaphor here, stepping over the cracks in the pavement is an act of detachment, dismissiveness, passiveness. In recent years, nature writing has become for me the kind of embodied tool that Leah Manaema Avene touches upon, helping to communicate and harness a deeper connection to the landscape within and outside myself. What draws me to nature writing as a practice is how you don't have to be an environmental scientist or know the name of every species of plant or animal in order to immerse yourself.

One key element of nature writing is observation, and it's here that I find myself in a meditative state, paying attention only to the micro: the army of caterpillars nibbling on a nettle leaf, the lichen growing a home on the bark of a birch tree, or the bee dancing across a rockery of lavender. It gives you the superpower of making time elastic, and wonder feel abundant. You don't have to be a thousand feet up a mountain to attune to this skill either. Some of the most mesmerising ecosystems I've found have come from observing life in the literal cracks in the concrete. Colonies of ants carrying scraps of food, worms burrowing into the ground, centipedes and woodlice scurrying with seemingly no real sense of direction, among the dandelions, nettles, cleavers, daisies and fungi that all somehow manage to make a thriving home in the centimetres of space between the hardness of the human-made. Suddenly, our relationship with the cracks, and therefore both nature and grief, becomes more intimate, relational.

Engaging with nature in this way has offered a creative, world-opening perspective in my exploration of grief. After all, the seasonal life cycle of the natural world teaches us that decomposition, deterioration, decay, sowing, blooming and rebirth are simply a routine fact of life. During spring of 2023, I attended a series of nature-writing workshops for women and gender-diverse people of colour, led by the radiant Dalbinder Kular. The workshops took place in Sheffield's General Cemetery, whose grounds, home to centuries of history, are undergoing renovations to transform the space into a site of creation in the present.

As a preface to each session, Dal acknowledged the convoluted relationships that we, as people of colour, may have with the cemetery, with nature and with grief. With a breathing exercise, she encouraged us to engage with the workshop at whatever intensity felt safe for us. She then read an invocation to bring us collectively into the space. 'Recognise the human, the more-than-human, the once-was human, the resting and the yet-to-be human,' Dal began, before naming some of the people of colour known to be buried in the cemetery. Next came an ode to the wilderness, 'calling in' species from nuthatch to treecreeper, cinnabar moth to pipistrelle bat, fox to stone, moss to elm: 'Thank you to all the beings of this space . . . Our Wild Cemetery. It belongs to us all. Let us begin.'[8]

Dal's invocation succeeded in grounding me in the possibilities of the workshop every time, enabling me to leave behind the dissociative anxiety I'd entered with. I'd attend these sessions nervously anticipating my inability to connect with the grief I had buried. In the first session, for example, I found I did very little writing. Unable to put pen to paper, I instead spent much of it talking to Kisha, a Peaks of Colour volunteer also taking part. She expressed her excitement for the session, how the cemetery made her feel rebellious and unruly, compelling her to explore the forbidden.

I, on the other hand, couldn't concentrate on Dal's writing prompts because I was so in my head about where to begin. I almost felt behind, like a child who'd missed a day of school. I was relieved, then, when Kisha invited me to join her on a tombstone, where we compared our differing relationships with grief. Kisha grew up in America, where open-casket funerals were the norm. Death wasn't hidden from her, and as a result she has an enviable ability to speak of and with her lost relatives. Not without sorrow, but with acceptance and love.

It was this intimacy of shared grief that invigorated me, as I sat mesmerised by the ways that pearly-headed snowdrops wove themselves around the crypts, life thriving in an earth contaminated with death. So when Dal urged us to write a poem inspired by the prompt 'Remember . . .', I found my once-empty notebook filled with pages upon pages of musings. In the final reading, we stood in a circle and spoke our words aloud to the cemetery. Mine read as follows:

Remember,
In conversation with the human and
non-human kin, grief is held
You can't grieve alone.

Remember,
To bury the grief only constructs a tomb for pain
You can't grieve alone.

Remember,
Grief is communal. A shared truth,
a collective inevitability
You can't grieve alone.

Remember,
Snowdrops bloom through the cracks of decay
You can't grieve alone.

My words felt like an instruction manual for how to navigate the road ahead. A reminder of my own needs, and of the truths that can so often get lost in the lies we tell ourselves. If my poem signified the start of this journey, however, Kisha's felt like a destination I longed to visit someday. She called in the tastes and aromas of the cultural dishes which reminded her of each family member she had lost. There was a tangible intimacy here to which I so wished I could edge closer. Yet by the final workshop, I had transformed my relationship with the cemetery. Once a foreboding place I associated with feeling intimidatingly inferior to during the day and, as a woman, unsafe at night, I reimagined it as a haven for nocturnal wildlife. A forbidden forest rave where, under the disco moon, the tawny owls, hares, foxes and moles would come out to cut shapes on the pine-needled dance floor.

Alongside this transformed sense of place, I also unlocked a connection with grief that I would never have been able to imagine three months prior. For this, I have Dal and the daffodil to thank. During one workshop we were challenged to find an item, or 'being' as Dal described it, among the cemetery grounds that we felt drawn towards. I instinctively chose a daffodil. It was a spring day that teased blue skies out from behind lingering clouds. For the past few months my body had felt enclosed, tightly moulded into a cocoon in an attempt to protect myself from the inevitability of seasonal depression. The meadows of daffodils reminded me to shake off the winter blues and stretch into the possibility of springtime. With this embodied hope in my chosen being, I found myself able to permeate the cracks in the layers of concrete laid over the buried relationships with myself, my grandma and with nature. Cracks that helped me feel slightly closer to what lies beneath.

'If you were to ask your being to introduce itself, what would it say?' Dal prompted, creating space for us to give voice to nature, before asking, 'What would your being witness of you now?' Through the compassionate voice of a daffodil, I imagined a conversation held between soon-to-bloom buds.

She needs us.
They whisper, turning to each other's blooming ears to conspire.

Each winter weighs heavier and she's forgetting who she is.
A tired bud agrees.

How do we know that she'll even appreciate us?
Grunts one, belligerently tightening its petals.

We help her remember, we help her connect to her namesake, and she repays us in heart smiles.
Came a firm rebuttal.

Pleading and plotting continued into the crisp spring night. And, in the morning, yellowed sunbeams had blossomed.

Despite feeling warmed with gratitude for these delicate yellow flowers, they also served as an uncomfortable reminder of who was still missing as the seasons changed. When I allow myself to think of my granny, I remember her in a lemon-yellow sailor's dress, which now hangs in the back of my wardrobe. I think of us hand in hand, trespassing across a disused football field in Doncaster, which sprung to life every spring. We'd make this journey to pick a posy of daffodils that we'd gift to my mum every Mother's Day.

Writing in nature allowed me to harness the power of storytelling to connect with this suppressed memory, and transform it into a commitment to embody the unconditional radiance that spring brings. I believe there will be something in nature that speaks to each of us in this way, and that might enable us to give voice to our grief.

Alongside these deep moments of personal growth, Dal's workshop spaces also helped me uncover a grief that I had not yet begun to name. I'd been preoccupied with the human losses that dominated my worldview, but what surfaced in these sessions was an acknowledgement too of ecological grief and a processing of the loss of my once favourite place.

Situated less than six miles from the centre of Sheffield, and accessible via a woodland trail, Rivelin Reservoir was the place that made this city feel like home for me. Living in my memory as hues of blues and greens, Rivelin existed as the colour palette of a peaceful soul and a calmed nervous system. Here, I'd experience a coming-home to myself that only took place when lying on my back, floating with arms outstretched in its bone-numbing waters. Time went by at the speed of clouds. An elastic time that gave permission for you to emerge having forgotten whatever pains had brought you to the shore in the first place.

Rivelin Reservoir, however, can now only be described as my 'former favourite place'. Over the past couple of years it has gradually been destroyed. First came the 'no swimming' and 'no trespassing signs'. Bold, red and garish, but easy to ignore. The eight-foot metal fences, however, demanded acknowledgement. An eyesore. When those of us prone to trespassing found we could actually utilise the fence to leverage ourselves over the neighbouring wall, barbed wire was installed. The closure of the car park and picnic area soon followed. Then came the raising of the water levels in an attempt to submerge the pebbled shores. The waters rose so high that inches of trees were also under water. That didn't matter though, because soon after they were felled. Towering red pines, Douglas firs and red cedars reduced to stumps. A once vibrant, tranquil lagoon was transformed into a construction site, successfully made so unappealing that even the most determined of wild swimmers, like myself, couldn't bear to witness the destruction of something once so loved. Hiring a groundskeeper, or even a lifeguard, would have been much cheaper.

It's been almost three years since I last found myself in Rivelin's waters, and the more I processed this severing from place, the more love I felt in my chest. I began to understand that in suppressing the grief for so long, I had unwittingly restrained so much potential for the quiet intimacies that come with being rooted in place. In *Braiding Sweetgrass*, Potawatomi botanist Robin Wall Kimmerer reminds us that within a capitalism that transforms us into the living dead, leaving us bereft, we must also grieve a land that could assist in our healing were we not so disconnected from it. Pouring her love for her wild home onto the page, she discusses the loss of land through settler colonialism – land as fundamental to an indigenous sense of self, identity, connection to ancestors, as home of their non-human kinfolk, pharmacy, library and sustenance. As she expands: 'Our lands were where our responsibility to the world was enacted, sacred ground. It belonged to itself; it was a gift, not a commodity, so it could never be bought or sold [...] And so – in the eyes of the federal government – that belief was a threat.'[9]

Settler colonialism entrenched the notion of land as property, capital, real estate and resource that is still perpetuated today. The forces of capitalism would much rather we pour concrete over the cracks of our grief than see them as open spaces of possibility through which we can connect with the deeper responsibilities we have to the land and to each other. Yet remembering and rebuilding, as Wall Kimmerer says, is a generational act of resistance in the face of such loss. Through nature connection I find myself a perpetual student of the ways we might all seek to nurture something, or someone, in grief and in love. Through my work with Peaks of Colour, and as an individual steward, the roles of weaver, healer, caregiver, builder and visionary intersect and overlap. And with the love of flora instilled in me by my grandma, I set out in earnest, unearthing ways in which the restoration of our communities and of the land can begin to be nourished, here in the Peak District.

Grief as a Canyon

I never bought into the Hallmark idea that when a heart breaks it does so neatly, zig-zagged lines splitting it evenly in two. Instead, the heart feels like more of a map which traces the loves and the losses of a life. Focus your gaze and instead of arteries and blood vessels you will find an undulating landscape, and we are but the cartographers, navigating its memories, yearnings, fears and sorrows. For so long, I've felt certain that a biopsy of my heart would expose a cartoon-like canyon, an almighty crack that was formed there many years ago – the first heartbreak striking like a rumbling earthquake across its foundations.

With each additional grief that followed, the crevice widened. On one side, a dusty landscape, barren except for rolling tumbleweeds. Grey clouds loom overhead, weighted with animosity. Perched on the echoing precipice of this canyon, however, I can see that way off in the distance the other side of my heart is flourishing. There are meadows carpeted with wildflowers and thriving vegetation and an abundance of ripe fruit hangs in orchards, which are home to a population of bees and butterflies, and birdsong. The possibility of eternal spring beams over the infinite chasm, an invitation prohibited only by lack of access. I've longed for a bridge of outstretched hands to reach across the void and carry me to the other side, but this canyon feels impossible to cross alone.

In *We, The Heartbroken*, her series of reflective essays, Gargi Bhattacharyya reframes grief as heartbreak, and asks us to reconsider our understanding of its potential for change. Describing this heartbrokenness as a necessary component of any transformative politic, she writes that this sorrow transcends individual grief and the consciousness of all that is broken in the world, all which must be mended. Grief, therefore, is a haunting that moves between private suffering and collective horror – and haven't we been surrounded by so much of that of late?

We are heartbroken, Bhattacharyya poses, not only because of loss, but because of knowledge too: 'Not only because life ends, but also because life disappoints. And, most of all, not only because into each life some rain must fall, but also because the deluge washing away the possibilities of human life sweeps down generations, reducing us all.'[10]

To ignore something of this magnitude can only corrode our sense of self, Bhattacharyya suggests, yet to find communion among such heartache repositions grief as the one common unifier. When harnessed correctly, a class consciousness – that is, a galvanising mode of collective knowledge – grounded in an emotion so powerful, could incite revolution. Our shared sadness is in fact a vital prelude to our resistance, 'the thing that makes it possible for us to see each other and the world and what has been and is being done to us all'.[11]

If heartbreak thins our skin, Bhattacharyya reasons, our openness to each other is a balm that strengthens it beyond the human instinct of suppression. The remaking of our world, therefore, is conditional on us being able to carve out space and time to mourn. In many ways, Peaks of Colour represents my attempt to build the viaduct I am so desperate for. The bridge that will allow myself, and others, to traverse from a state of ruinous loss to the revolutionary grief and place of possibility that Bhattacharyya prophesies.

I've found that the beautiful thing about adopting a lived-experience and trauma-led approach to organising is that in creating a space that I need, it's likely that the space will be one that the community needs too. A walkshop Peaks of Colour co-curated in collaboration with Right to Roam organiser Nadia Shaikh did just that. It was called 'Grieving Lost Possibilities' and saw a group of people of colour build ourselves a home for grief in the rolling valleys of Edale.

The first workshop was led by writer and founder of Feminist Invoicing Monika Radojevic, whose gentle guidance supported us to reckon with the uncomfortable but necessary reminder that we can't heal from what we avoid, suppress or minimise. As the river gurgled in the background, she guided us to write invoices to the white supremacy and the patriarchy for all that disconnects us from ourselves, each other and the land. One person invoiced capitalism for their inability to rest, another for memories of a lost loved one whose happiness in old photographs they'd no longer be able to experience, another for the magic lost alongside thousands of species now extinct. It was a creative and disruptive way of repurposing the invoice, an arguably mundane tool of capitalism and bureaucracy, into a template with which to quantify our traumas, process losses and better understand what we're owed from a society that perpetually takes.

Throughout the day clouds passed overhead, inquisitive sheep inspected our goings-on and stoneflies danced around us. By lunch it was clear that this place had become something of a haven. The river made a gurgling border for our grief as the afternoon continued, helping us to enclose it for safekeeping with the gentle guidance of Healing Justice London founder Farzana Khan. As the session drew to a close, Farzana led us to the water. On either side of the river we formed lines facing one another, and each let go of one of the bereavements that weighed heavy for us. I set free 'avoidance' as a comfortable survival strategy that kept me safe, once, but no longer served me. Together, we watched as the river carried our innermost demons away.

Our burnout roars most ferociously when we are consumed by the impossibility of our pasts, presents and futures combined. Gifting your losses to the earth, its waters, fires and soils, may seem frivolous amid such abject horror. However, finding opportunities such as these – no matter how temporary – to let go of elements of our grief quells the embers of yesterday that ignite in us when we feel most vulnerable. This is how we build our capacity for rest.

In that little corner of the Peak District we made a home for ourselves that was so encompassing, it was easy to forget that a world full of financial woes, work stress, childcare, deadlines and never-ending chores even existed. As we followed the familiar route back, I was struck by the variety of the losses that came up for people in that space across the day. While many of us processed the more tangible losses of loved ones, one person grieved the self that was lost when they had a child, another the dualities of past, present and future selves that arose when transitioning. I grieved the person I could have been had it not been for abusive partners stealing my opportunity to be defined as anything other than a survivor or a victim. These personal instances of grief had been held in a communal experience so unlike the individualised grieving we are otherwise offered as a way forwards, and together we let them go.[12] As Bhattacharyya suggests, our survival, if we are to have it at all, must be through togetherness.

The seeds for this event were first sown a year prior, during a Peaks of Colour sound-bathing walkshop, co-facilitated by the infectious Muna McAdie. For so long my grief had felt opaque. I have pictures of the people I've lost in albums stored on my phone and in framed pictures around my house, yet I'd never look directly at them. I'd become adept at unseeing and unfeeling. When I tried to think of my grandparents, I could see their outlines, their clothes – her daffodil-yellow dress with the white sailor collar, and his mauve bomber jacket and tweed trilby hat. But I could never see their faces.

Yet lying down in an orchard, situated in the grounds of a woodland community centre, I saw them both in my mind's eye for the first time in over fifteen years. My grandad stood in the doorway of their tiny kitchen, leaning on the frame just as he used to, observing the family filling the walls of his two-up two-down terraced house. My grandma, bouncy silver hair fresh from her rollers, pottered about around him, floating in and out between the door frame, turning her back as she washed the pots, bending down to feed one of her many, many cats, then floating through the doorway again, into the living room, just out of shot. It was a fleeting moment that lasted a lifetime.

In this scene I was only an observer. I couldn't communicate with them, touch them. I had a sense that if I averted my gaze in any way, I'd lose their image forever. When eventually the melodic bass of the gong pulled me away from the scene, I felt as if my legs were being forced to walk backwards, despite desperately wanting to stay in my grandparents' living room. From there, with Muna's sonic guidance, I drifted into a light sleep. By the time the session finished and I opened my eyes, I realised I'd been crying. The first tears shed for either grandparent since their respective passings. As my vision returned, I saw a community of people of colour yawn and stretch themselves back into the present, and while I sat with the surrealness of my experience, I felt held. It was a reminder that we don't have to wade our way through even the most personal of losses alone, that there are embodied ways of travelling through grief, and that it is possible to find bridges back to ourselves and the ones we love. They've just been hidden from us for too long.

What I now know to be true is that grief weighs lighter when held in community, and lighter still when that community is held in nature. Finding or forging spaces such as these is a radical prerogative. A revolutionary opportunity. A second sight. A home-grown infrastructure for healing. When we open ourselves up to the possibilities of heartbreak, we are able to build bridges of community care over canyons of pain, bridges that allow us to dance between the dark and the light more freely. We're able to grow our own medicine in the cracks of despair, medicine that allows us to have agency to attend to our wounds. We're able to create beautifully imperfect works of art out of our own brokenness, a brokenness transformed into lives affirmed. For so long I have felt powerless, rooted in self-pity, vulnerable, at the behest of a trauma-tising world. But as Gargi Bhattacharyya reminds us, at the heart of all revolutionary consciousness is collective heartbreak: 'How can it not be? Who can imagine another world unless they have already been broken apart by the world we're in?'[13]

On Radical Rage

Black rage in an anti-black world is a spiritual virtue ...
Rage is the public cry for black dignity ... Rage is the
work of love that stands against an unloving world.
— Danté Stewart[1]

A ngry. A stereotype that has followed Black people for decades. Malcolm X, Michelle Obama, Serena Williams, Oprah, Will Smith. No matter how talented, how respected, how professional, how skilled we may be in our respective fields, it is likely that an animalistic caricature of ourselves will be weaponised against us the moment we dare to express anything close to frustration. Righteous as our rage may be, 'Angry Black' is a prefix that forms in the mouths of others as a given, blurring the lines between self and self-expression in those familiar phrases 'Angry Black woman' or 'Angry Black man'. Yet where does our anger end and our Blackness begin? It's a question that is made all the harder to answer given the decades of emotional suppression that has arisen in response to this trope.

This has created internalised fear among Black communities to such an extent that in our decades-long attempt to reject both the stereotype and its consequences, we have learned to subdue our anger, to turn away from the human need to release an emotion only natural in the face of oppression. The most shameful of emotions, suppressed and neglected, that gurgling, spitting, bubbling rage only builds with every microaggression, racial slur, political injustice and shouldered harm, until one day something, a mild inconvenience perhaps, causes this rage to overflow.

A self-combusting burning ball of fire that consumes us and everyone we touch until we eventually burn out. A stereotype realised.

That so much of our work in activist spaces is fuelled by this
anger makes it worthy of study here. Movements and revolutions
have been built upon a fury ablaze, and while this may appear
like a productive channelling of emotion on the surface, without
intentional care our anger will engulf us, reducing our flames
to embers. Approaching our rage with intentionality, therefore,
challenges a perception of what a restful revolution should look
and feel like. Though soft in its handling of our exhaustion, and
gentle in its holding of our grief, we do not want to lie down and
make a comfortable bed with our anger. Instead of submitting to it,
internalising it perhaps, the release of anger we so desperately seek
requires our postures of rest to contort into something beautiful.

Rage as a Melodic Posture

In a keynote presentation delivered at Connecticut's National
Women's Studies Association Conference in June 1981, Audre
Lorde read from an essay titled 'The Uses of Anger: Women
Responding to Racism'. In it she asserts that the only logical way
we can respond to the indignity of racism is through anger. Global
majority people, particularly women of colour, Lorde tells us, 'have
grown up with a symphony of anger, [...] knowing that when
we survive, it is in spite of a world that takes for granted our lack
of humanness, and which hates our very existence outside of its
service.'[2] Her choice of 'symphony' rather than 'cacophony' is significant here, she tells us, as we need to come to a place where we
might 'orchestrate those furies' rather than let them destroy us.

'Mad' by Solange Knowles is a melodic exploration of forbidden anger written by an artist who I repeatedly return to in times
of crisis. It can quite aptly be described as a symphony of anger.

Beckoning the listener to do just as Lorde instructs – to listen to anger's rhythms, then to excavate its power beyond its mere presentation – Solange refuses to be silenced by fear. Instead, she revels in the ethereal beauty of Black rage and validates our vulnerabilities by reminding us that exploring our anger, making peace with it and setting it free is an act of self-love. She is a woman in control. Yet the floating melodic delivery of 'Mad' also conveys a woman who's weary – too tired to shout or yell or scream. Throughout the song, Solange enters a recurring conversation with a critical other, who repetitively asks why she's always got to be so mad. Solange's response remains the same. And by the final lines, Solange tells her listeners how draining it is to be constantly explaining and justifying her feelings. There is a defeatism here that speaks to the ways that burnout festers in the rotting wounds of untapped or misunderstood anger.

'Mad' is the sixth track on Solange's Grammy award-winning third studio album *A Seat at the Table*. The album's impact rippled through the consciousness of the Black imagination, with audiences feeling seen and heard in the softness of Black emotionality. I was one such listener. In fact, *A Seat at the Table* resonated with me so deeply that I have the album cover tattooed on my right ankle. It's a compilation of songs that evoke the tenderness of a lullaby, and pieces such as 'Mad' soothe me when I need to feel understood, to find belonging, when I need to be reminded that these emotions are bigger than me and that I'm not alone in them. That we have a lot to be mad about. It's a song that forces a reckoning with all the infuriating moments of harm and injustice that have been left unaddressed.

As a Black domestic abuse survivor, for example, I was never allowed to express my anger at what was being done to me. If I was anything other than obedient, I would face a strangling or, worse, silent treatment. I packaged all the wrath that was left unexpressed in the moments where I couldn't fight back and boxed them into dark crevices of my brain, among the other dusty hoarded horrors. Soon these attics began to overflow, and I reasoned that to build a home for the rage in the brick and mortar that are my bones and flesh was the safest form of concealment. Anger, embodied.

It's for this reason that anger is still the least addressed emotion I carry, and the one I feel the most shame about. I don't think I'm alone in either of these things. So many of us deny our anger or hate ourselves for it. It's the anger of my teenage years that brings me the most guilt, however. I don't quite remember what I did during those blinding fits of adolescent rage, when, with no viable outlet, the layers of grief and self-loathing had solidified. But I think it was an anger that made my little brother afraid of me or resentful of me, or both. It was an anger that caused my mum to say, 'You're just like your dad' on more than one occasion. An anger that indented the dashboard of her old Nissan Micra. An anger that I would take out on myself with razor blades. An anger that I would quickly learn to repress, but which has now been neglected for so long that I can barely access it. An anger that only resurfaces at the sign of injustice.

A Seat at the Table was released in 2017. With 'I've got a lot to be mad about' echoing in my brain throughout that time, I was able to consider the weight of the resentments that I had collected over the years. The list spanned pages upon pages in a notebook – some lines of which are relayed opposite, where it's received something of an update. The anger doesn't go away, after all. It just evolves. So many of us will have a song that speaks for us in ways we couldn't express ourselves. Writing it out like this – as lyrics dragged across the page – was, for me, a visual way of bringing that hidden rage reverberating to the surface.

I've Got a Lot to be Mad About

Saw my skin, brown, Black, Rendered me voiceless. Turned me Black and Blue.

I'm mad at the white men who beat me. Strangled me. Raped me. Twisted my brain into knots. Cheated and cheated and cheated and cheated.

as a vulnerability to be exploited or fetish to be enjoyed. Made me their plaything, Rendered me

I'm mad at the white men – and women – in police uniforms who dismissed me. Who believed his fabricated defence,

and, upon giving my abuser a warning, said 'I'm a good judge of character, he seems an alright guy'.

I'm mad at the white institutions that profit off my pain. Year after year, I pay to heal from the actions of

white men,

Reinforcing a narrative, that I'm the crazy one in this relationship, the fear of

not being believed silences the anger that could free us.

A.C.A.B

Who prosper on the reparations and accountability I am owed. The Survivor's Tax.

Rage as a Liberatory Posture

Audre Lorde reminds us that our anger has ensured our survival thus far, so before we give it up we must find a practice that can take its place. While writing has been one of the mediums that brings my pain to the surface, I'm yet to find an avenue to release it and set it free. It's for this reason that I wanted to speak to someone who has found their outlet, and a friend suggested Venus. Despite having not met in person before, we immediately feel at ease when we meet on Zoom. I'm in bed, wearing a hoodie and with a hot water bottle soothing period pains, and Venus is taking out her braids. It feels right that a discussion on the hardest of emotions should be cushioned with such softness. We talk about the shame and guilt that comes from harbouring unprocessed anger and the instances of violence this is rooted in.

'Being a sex worker, and someone who does martial arts, is an interesting experience. It's almost like people assume that the strength of the latter cancels out the vulnerability of the other,' Venus begins. 'I consider myself to be a survivor of many types of harm, but it's often perceived that I can't be victimised because I'm "strong" or "confident" or whatever.'

As the founder of Sex and Rage (an organisation led by sex workers, educators and activists) and the former co-founder of Shadow Sistxrs Fight Club (which ran martial arts and self-defence classes for QTIBIPOC and FLINTA [female, lesbian, intersex, trans and agender] communities), Venus is a self-described 'professional afrodisiac'. She tells me that her anger, once invisible and internalised like my own, manifested as passivity in the face of the rage of others: 'Regardless of what kind of sex work you do, people will often project their own anger on to you,' she explains. 'This projected anger is embodied, so our solution to it must be too. That's why a big part of my healing has been allowing myself to get angry and upset, to not suppress it.'

This sense of an embodied practice – of emotion transformed into the physical and visible – is foundational to Venus's work, a tool to redirect anger into something that is healing, as opposed to harmful. 'It's an alchemical process that makes us feel powerful. It's an invaluable skill that allows us to firstly keep ourselves physically safe against so much racialised, sexualised violence, but secondly it offers a psychological, somatic release of so many emotions.' I tell her I envy this and describe a 'boxing for mental health' class in Sheffield that I haven't been able to bring myself to go to. It's run only by white men, I tell Venus, and the thought of them witnessing me in the rage other white men have caused makes me feel too uncomfortable to go. 'See, I grew up around martial arts,' Venus tells me. 'In the eighties my dad was karate world champion, my mum was the English karate champion, so I was always around a racially diverse community of fighters.'

'It wasn't until my friend Bones – an artist and performer – invited me to facilitate a session, that I realised I'd been taking this for granted,' she explains, 'that it should be shared. This is how my work with Shadow Sistxrs came to be.' She groans, tugging at a tightly woven braid that is proving difficult to unplait. 'Around the same time, I was also questioning with my partner – who is not a sex worker – and others, asking: How do we create a space that's embodied, empowering, safe? That prioritises sex workers, and that also allows people who are not sex workers to learn and support in a way that isn't exploitative? This is how Sex and Rage came to be. As the name suggests, it's offering sexual liberation as a tool for processing and making sense of these big feelings like rage. To allow the often contradictory and conflicting experiences you may have to be expressed, without shame.'

Much of Venus's work unabashedly uses the language of rage and fighting. It's interesting to me that this would traditionally evoke negative connotations, but by offering practices which allow us to redefine and reclaim our rage, Venus is challenging that narrative. Beyond this, she also demonstrates the ways that the fluid sensuality of erotic acrobatics or the disciplined poise of a swinging high kick can be adopted as new postures. Postures that can be experimented with as we move towards a restful revolution.

Rage as a Defiant Posture

The more traditional posture that immediately springs to mind when I consider anger, however, is one of resistance. Of a sea of people, feet pummelling the concrete in unison, backs straight, heads proud, eyes focused, and fists raised defiantly into the sky. From the Black Panthers to the 1968 Olympics, Nelson Mandela to the Black Lives Matter uprisings of 2020, throughout history, the salute has become an emblem of Black Power, of our hurt and rage transformed into solidarity and action. 'We only have to look around us to see how anger is the primary motivator for change. It's not an undirected, wayward anger, it's not a tantrum,' Venus explains. 'It's very channelled and controlled, poignant and well-defined. There are tangible, concrete reasons why that anger exists. It starts by being angry at the persecution, the lack of safety, the discrimination, the exclusion, the lack of opportunity, the victimisation. And then it becomes something more than anger, it becomes a form of transformative justice.'

This rings true across liberation struggles. Before Pride became co-opted into a consumerist street party-cum-festival, for example, it originated as a march to commemorate the Stonewall riots – which arose in response to the police raids of queer spaces and is now considered the catalyst for the LGBTQ+ rights movement which followed. Though the misconception that anger is synonymous with violence causes many to consider protests as undemocratic and irrational, they are how oppressed communities have been able to express our rage safely. The legacy of such protests shows how our anger can prevent us from becoming resigned to defeatism, and instead mobilise a demand for change.

Yet, as of 2020, the right to protest, enshrined in human rights law,[3] has been all but overturned in the UK, overshadowed by the Police, Crime, Sentencing and Courts (PCSC) Act. A Draconian law which brings with it fascist implications of state control, the PCSC was introduced as a reaction to the increasing momentum of gender, climate and racial justice activists during 2020. As a result, the act denies people the opportunity to resist the ever-increasing oppressions of the British state, while strengthening police power to dictate how we should conduct our protests and the severity of punishment for going against this.

The act ultimately ensures that protesters are effectively treated in the same vein as domestic terrorists. An individual protester may be fined up to £2,500, while anyone who causes damage to, for example, memorials could face up to *ten years* in prison. For context, the longest sentence usually given to a rapist is eight years. Not satisfied with these punishing restrictions, the Public Order Bill was then instated just one year later, with the intention of *preventing* 'serious disruption' – arguably the core objective of protests. Police now don't have to wait for serious disruption to happen; they can simply shut down a protest if they think it might occur. As a result, 'locking on' has been criminalised, suspicionless stop-and-searches are undertaken, and Serious Disruption Prevention Orders are issued to ban individuals from protesting.

The existence of the PCSC and Public Order Bill reveals both the power of collective anger to foster fear in our oppressors, and the staggering speed with which carceral controls can be tightened. In restricting our ability to protest, the state not only removes a vital tool of change from our communities, but also steals our ability to begin healing decades of intergenerational anger. For when we are made to turn away from protest, what's being denied is the transformation of anger into power. It is here that I currently find myself, peering into the possibilities held within my own vulner-abilities. It's nerve-wracking, and humbling. Yet, trusting in the process, I once again find myself turning to 'Mad' for inspiration.

When I saw Solange live at Lovebox festival[4] in 2017, I cried throughout the whole set. With my brother giving me regular side glances to check in, rubbing my shoulders and drawing me into a hug when he could see me sinking into my feelings a little too uncontrollably, bearing witness to the performance felt like an out-of-body experience. When she sang 'Mad', a portal of oranges, reds and purples pulsated like a sunset at the back of the stage. Though her previous performances had been lively, with synchro-nised choreography that saw her and her dancers moving as one, 'Mad' inspired a more mellow delivery. As she stood among her dancers, Solange's movements vibrated to a pause. Their bodies remained motionless as she sang, with only slight sporadic move-ments as if they were uncontrollable responses to certain lines. This all changed, however, when the lyrics began calling the audi-ence back to love as the solution to anger, a refrain whispering a repetitive reminder with increasing urgency. With each rising octave, the bodies upon the stage burst into life. As the postures of those on stage contorted and entwined, weaving among the reverberations, we received a somatic message that was clear: find a loving relationship with anger.

Rage as a Loving Posture

When we understand the power of our anger, we no longer need to fear it, or resent it. Suddenly, the most shameful of emotions becomes one we can make peace with, and finding ways to release this anger becomes how we show ourselves love, how we love each other. The writer and Buddhist teacher Lama Rod Owens explores how we can build a loving relationship with our anger in his book *Love and Rage: The Path of Liberation Through Anger.* Here, Owens speaks to the ways he, as a Black man, was conditioned to relate to his rage as something dangerous that would result in his own erasure through imprisonment or death. In exploring anger, however, he posits that this emotion derives from hurt, from a heartbrokenness that has been left unaddressed. When attended to with love for the self, however, he suggests that this grief and anger can transform into wisdom, and it's in this wisdom that we will find liberation. But as with everything else, we have to practise. There can be no liberation without it, he says.

Owens introduces readers to what he has termed the Seven Homecomings. Three of the Seven Homecomings are rooted in Buddhist teachings: The Guide (Buddha), The Wisdom Text (Dharma) and Community, as traditional sources of refuge. Expanding on this, he includes Ancestors, The Earth, Silence and Ourselves as grounding him 'in an expression of love that forms a container to hold the intensity of anger and rage'.[5] I'm not too proud to recognise that my ability to embrace my anger is in its infancy. Owen's framework of the Seven Homecomings shows this to be true: I don't currently feel able to attend to all the refuges he speaks of, and I'm sure others feel similarly. With Peaks of Colour's work rooted in both the Earth and Community, however, these are the two I find myself instinctively leaning towards. Owens says a big part of his practice is to reflect 'on the places, groups, and communities where [he] feels loved',[6] and so, in our walkshops, I too have begun to pay attention to the ways these two refuges entwine naturally as both an individual and collective practice.

Throughout 2023 and 2024, for example, Decolonising Economics founders Guppi Bola and Noni Makuyana brought together activists and artists doing radical work to connect, rest and conspire in a series of 'Nourishing Economics' retreats. The first was in the Derbyshire Dales, and despite wanting to focus all my energy on the retreat, I found myself distracted by an email that had caught my attention. It was from a white-led organisation that was removing funding from Peaks of Colour, despite previous assurances of financial security. In a moment our now un-funded organisation was plummeted into uncertainty. Yet while this was terrifying, it was the nonchalant way in which this information had been relayed that I really found infuriating. The incompetency of this organisation sent us back to square one, yet this email also used the delivery style of a housemate letting you know they'd forgotten to pick up the milk. *Oops!*

I felt the familiar warmth of injustice rise on the back of my neck as I read. It was an acidic, belching range that twists the pit of your stomach into a fiery knot, and after a few deep breaths I began crafting my venomous reply. As my fingers hovered hesitantly over the send button, I remembered Lorde's invocation. That we cannot and should not hide our anger to assuage the guilt of our oppressors. If we do, it risks becoming trivialised. If I were not to press send, this inflamed injustice would fester within me. The billionth injustice of its kind, pulling tighter and tighter at my chest. And, because I am no longer in the business of denigrating my own or my collaborators' efforts, I pressed send. Since dubbed the 'Email of All Emails' by another Decolonising Economics participant, this message represented Peaks of Colour's scary, thrilling, nerve-wracking and downright daft first attempt at unshackling ourselves from the chains of professionalism. And it was liberating.

After sending, I shut my laptop and went to join the Decolonising Economics workshops. Light-headed and feeling slightly empty, I was vibrating from the sickening sensation that I was about to introduce myself to a group of new friends after having done something so character-changing that I barely knew who I was. As I led the group on a ramble the next day, I still felt unsettled, almost like the new relationships I was making were being built on dishonesty. It was here, nestled at the foot of a tumbling weir, that I shared the Email of All Emails with my new-found community. It was a message that everyone in the Derbyshire Dales that week wished they could have sent at some point, if not multiple points, in their organising. And as one of our glorious comrades, Jumoke, gathered us in a circle and offered a dramatic reading of my lengthy rebuttal, gasps, whoops and mm-hmms of solidarity erupted from the circle. As the words carried in the breeze we laughed at the absurdity, the audacity, of such a response, and I no longer felt alone in my rage.

This was a new experience for me. To share my anger, my most vulnerable of emotions, and have it not only validated but celebrated was overwhelmingly humbling. I felt the love from each and every single person in that space, yet I still didn't feel quite right. Before I had a chance to make sense of this, Asma, a friend and fellow Sheffielder, stepped forward. With an infectious energy, she said, 'Shall we all scream?' Within moments, she had lined us up along the riverbank, and after counting us down from three, led us in an almighty scream. A choir of activists erupting in a chorus of collective rage. It echoed in the sunken valley, before being drowned out by the voluminous sounds of the weir. Our rage, captured and held by the love we shared for each other, and the earth.

Following the Email of All Emails, we incorporated 'unprofessionalism' into Peaks of Colour's core principles. Maintaining the transformative-justice ethos of 'do no harm', I realised that unprofessionalism gives us permission to reject collectively the pressure to be palatable, likeable, reasonable and measured in the face of harm and violence. An abject rejection of respectability politics, it allows us to resist the conditioned impulse to bury anger under polite smiles and emails that begin with 'no worries'. As the Nourishing Economics community and I completed our walk that day, with fellow member June playing Rihanna's 'Bitch Better Have My Money' loud from a large speaker, I knew this to be true. I experienced what it means to be able to speak our minds, name the injustice, point to the hypocrisy and express unequivocally how we are impacted, before walking away feeling confident that we're leaving a situation with as much resolution as we can source for ourselves.

At its core, Peaks of Colour aims to introduce our communities to nature as a playground in which we can connect, imagine, heal. Over the years, however, our interactions with the 'outdoor sector' (which often sits within the charity industrial complex) have made it clear that the land that should be free to all is accessible only on the condition that we play by a diversifying rulebook. Our powerlessness thrives off our professionalism. As a result, any opportunity for us to reclaim a relationship with the land in our own vision is suppressed, and the righteous anger we feel subsequently is silenced. Our togetherness, however, takes the loneliness of our individual furies and unites us in a loving rage, ensuring that our screams for justice will never be silenced.

Rage as a Relational Posture

Immy Kaur is the co-founder and director of Civic Square, an organisation that explores how to create and co-build neighbourhoods that are ecologically safe, socially just and regenerative. When I spoke to her about anger and burnout, she echoed how a sense of communality is something that can in itself work as the antithesis to burnout: 'Unequivocally the thing that doesn't contribute to burnout at all is when I'm in flow with a group of people that are collectively and equitably sharing the labour, that are respecting and championing each other's skills, where I feel like we're moving some of the hoarded resource into justice work, future work,' she says.

What I was struck by when I met Immy, both in person and during our Zoom conversation, was her animated anger at the ways structural injustice impacts us so intimately. I recognise this as being a source of so much of my own rage too, and asked Immy if she thought it was an accurate observation in her own experiences working in Civic Square. She nodded. 'It's funny because I'm such a high-energy, high-gratitude, high-joy kind of person. I truly believe we can all do something, and I try to do everything I can too. So, anger isn't an emotion I'd necessarily associate with my being, except when it comes to the fucking system. When it comes to the commodification, the individualisation of this work, the lack of resourcing, the fact that the wider economy contributes to burnout and the other ways our bodies are unwell, yeah, I'm angry about that.'

When we spoke previously, Immy had been clear about a key demographic she felt needed to be held accountable for their contribution to this injustice: white women. She believes, and I agree, that white feminism (which is preoccupied exclusively with the needs of and issues impacting white, middle-class women, and seeks to attain an 'equality' defined as the same socio-political status as white men through carceral, capitalist means that rely on the continual subjugation of oppressed communities) has got a lot to answer for when it comes to the ways women and people of colour experience burnout.

'I have found white women in movement spaces hold unbelievably high standards for us in this work. Yet there is never a systematic analysis that recognises why we are not able to operate the way they think we should, or why we don't want to,' Immy explains. 'For generations white women have upheld structures that ensure we are perpetually under-resourced, and overworked, and then, when we do burn out, white women will be the first to weaponise it to delegitimise us. In one breath they will say, "You're not doing enough, you're not doing this, you're not doing that," then when we burn ourselves out trying to meet these unrealistic cultural and structural standards, they use our burnout to evidence that our work, racial justice work, isn't doable. There's actually a lot of people who don't want us doing this work, and they create systems so impenetrable that navigating them causes us to burn out.'

There's something sadistic about this cycle of burnout and rage. The way our anger drives us to do this work, only then to be packaged into a system that firstly causes us to burn out, before using our burnout to undermine our work, and therefore anger, all over again. History illustrates how white women have been instrumental in the weaponsiation of their whiteness against racialised communities. In *They Were Her Property: White Women as Slave Owners in the American South*, for example, Stephanie Jones-Rogers' extensive research into the archival history of the antebellum South evidences the depth of white women's involvement in the economic institution of slavery. Through the testimonies of enslaved people, reinforced by an array of narrative sources, legal and financial documents, military and government correspondence, she found that 'white southern women and girls knew the most obnoxious features of slavery all too well.

Slave-owning women and girls not only witnessed the most brutal features of slavery, they took part in them, profited from them and they defended them.[7]

Similarly, in *White Tears/Brown Scars: How White Feminism Betrays Women of Color*, Ruby Hamad documents the social involvement of white women during slavery. 'White women were integral to this spectacle of violence,' she says, 'encouraged to attend lynchings, which often had the atmosphere of family picnics. Women can be seen smiling in many of the postcards that were fashioned from the gruesome scenes and sold for a dime a dozen in corner stores. Images show mangled black bodies burned alive or hanging from trees while white people swarm around mugging for the camera.'[8]

The subjugation of Black Americans continued to be upheld by white women long after slavery too. The lynching of Emmett Till, for example, is a loss that still reverberates through generations of Black consciousness today. A fourteen-year-old boy from Chicago, Emmett was visiting family in Mississippi during the summer of 1955. While he was in a convenience store, he was accused by a white woman, Carolyn Bryant, of whistling at her. Carolyn's husband, along with a mob of white men, subsequently abducted Emmett and tortured him to death. They then dumped his body in the Tallahassee River, where he was found days later. With the support of Carolyn's testimony, the killers were acquitted by an all-white jury.

Though it is people of colour who find themselves with 'angry' as a descriptor of our personhood, Hamad highlights white women's conscious understanding of their power to manipulate their own anger – and systems of harm such as policing – against racialised communities. One such example is the 'damsel in distress' archetype. Now more colloquially known as 'Karens' in popular culture, the damsel in distress ensures their own protection at the expense of another's victimisation. Despite relegating themselves to a subordinate status in the process, 'the damsel in distress' is defined by their racial and sexual purity and innocence. A clear example of this took place in 2020 when Christian Cooper, a Black man, was out birdwatching in Central Park. He asked a white woman, Amy Cooper, to put her dog on a lead as is required by the park's rules, but when she erupted in outrage he captured it on his phone and posted on social media.

'I'm going to tell them there's an African American male threatening my life,' she says, before proceeding to call the police twice, firstly telling them, 'I'm being threatened by a man in the Ramble. Please send the cops immediately,' then accusing him of assault, which she later admitted was untrue. She was charged with one misdemeanour count of falsely reporting an incident and consequently lost her job. Hamad describes Amy Cooper's actions as both damaging and violent, something which the district attorney also recognised in a statement about the case, which read: 'fortunately no one was injured or killed in the police response to Ms Cooper's hoax.'[9]

Beyond its manipulation of the public sphere, white feminism has also found a professional home in organising spaces such as those that Immy and I work within. Audre Lorde has been specific in naming the violence perpetrated by white women in such spaces as something that fuels her own anger. Reeling off a bullet-pointed list of examples, she cites quotes overheard and received from white women engaging with racial justice work:

'Tell me how you feel but don't say it too harshly or I cannot hear you,' said one.

'I think I've gotten a lot. I feel Black women really understand me a lot better now; they have a better idea of where I'm coming from,' reflected another.

'It allows me to deal with racism without dealing with the harshness of Black women.'

The list goes on.

One place I have seen this unfold most viciously is in the VAWG sector. Despite being victims of patriarchal harm in interpersonal relationships themselves, many women in positions of power are using the same patriarchal tactics of power, control, coercion and manipulation against the most marginalised of survivors and their allies.[10] Calling themselves 'gender-critical feminists' – also known by their critics as TERFs (trans-exclusionary radical feminists) or, as I prefer, fascist feminists – their institutional status is wielded to distort gendered-violence services through a radicalised anti-trans agenda.

Targeting trans and gender-non-conforming survivors of domestic abuse and sexual violence, this aggression – perpetrated under the guise of 'feminism' – is nothing short of a campaign of hate in which, once again, the anger of white cis women is weaponised. Gender-expansive communities have become a convenient scapegoat for the anger these women feel at their own victimisation and powerlessness, relentless still, despite having relied on a carceral system that rarely delivers on the promise of healing and justice. They are protected by racial, gendered and class privilege and concerned only with their own comfort and security under capitalism, and women and people of colour's ability to rest is then negligible and negotiable.

As a result, we see women's services unapologetically excluding trans survivors from their support, while CEOs and trustee boards lobby local councils and national governments to remove the basic human rights of a demographic of people who are disproportionately at risk of multiple forms of harm. With a national shortage of LGBT+ services available, trans survivors often have nowhere else to go but return to the abuse that gender-critical feminists purport to be so against. 'White women's work has material, physical, life-threatening consequences on people's lives. The conflict that it creates within our movements is also devastating,' Immy considers. 'We should be building solidarity, we should be supporting each other, we should be generous with each other, we should be learning together, learning from mistakes together. Our movements are relational, but this system has sowed the seeds of division and conflict and competition. It pits people against each other. It's quite perverse, voyeuristic almost. White women ask us to speak truth to power then use their power to protect the systems that we tell them are hurting us.'

When I consider the bubbling rage of injustice that so many of us are carrying, I imagine a scene with rows of statuesque individuals frozen in the hardening implications of their own anger. These people inhabit postures of violence, of an abusive partner lunging for the neck of their next victim, of a crumpled teenager whose wrist sits below a razor blade poised between their forefinger and thumb, of a scowling funder sat upon the pile of cash that is lorded over communities, or of a white woman wielding her phone as a weapon. When we start to attend to our collective rage, however, we can attune ourselves to the ways it teaches us our boundaries, identifies our triggers, reveals our needs and offers many different forms beyond the abandonment of ourselves, or each other. To begin posturing towards a restful resistance could look like bodies moving to the rhythms of their own music, like the freedom of personal sexual expression, like feet planted firmly into the soil in the position of battle, like clenched fists raised to the sky in protest, like mouths open wide bringing forth the release of an almighty scream, or like the many ways we come together in community to create change. In each posture, we are reminded: none of us can be free until all of us are free.

Case Study #2: Education

There is no such thing as a neutral educational process. Education either functions as an instrument which is used to facilitate integration of the younger generation into the logic of the present system and bring about conformity, or it becomes the practice of freedom, the means by which [people] deal critically and creatively with reality and discover how to participate in the transformation of their world.

— Paulo Freire[1]

In continuing to trace the origins of our burnout to the institutions that facilitate it, an exploration of our education systems feels fitting. It is the classroom, after all, that dominates so much of our time during childhood, and that moulds our personal, professional and political sense of self. Our schools *should* be a place of nourishment and enrichment: where we are given the freedom to experiment, be curious and creative; where learning is presented to us as the ability to follow new paths; where an understanding of our place in, and responsibility to, the wider social and environmental landscape is nurtured. In this second case study, however, I explore how instead schools are so often where we learn much of the conditionings of a capitalist system that prime us for burnout in adult life.

Across the West, the expansive potential of education is being suppressed, with the sweeping rejection of critical consciousness within curriculums. In the USA, critical race theory (CRT) – the study of race and racism as a socio-political and socio-economic construct – has been banned across the country, with anti-CRT measures introduced across forty-nine states, and secondary schools being the most targeted. Here, compliance is compulsory, with one in three measures withholding funding from schools as a consequence of violations.[2]

Meanwhile, the UK's curriculum has never included our racial history, and the enduring legacy of Empire and British involvement in the slave trade has yet to be represented truthfully. In 2021, a petition signed by over 200,000 people called for this to change, something the then-schools minister Nick Gibb rejected. 'It risks lowering educational standards,' he said. 'The danger is that it does detract from that professional normal autonomy, and it is that professional autonomy that is driving up standards.'[3] This erasure of history in order not to disrupt the capitalist status quo is a tried-and-tested colonial strategy that ensures generation upon generation are denied a true embodied knowing of self and society in service of a capitalist labour market. Lost among this duality of belonging and unbelonging, we burn out.

Education as Capitalist Conditioning

To recognise the myths of education under capitalism, we can look to previous generations' experiences as a compass. Ola Fagbohun, for example, is an equitable aging consultant, coach, researcher and the founder of The Zest OF:

You Project, a Sheffield-based organisation which supports peri- and post-menopausal people in racialised communities to navigate ageing, health and wellbeing. 'It's easy to paint the past as nothing but suffering, but the reality is, Black children navigating education during the seventies and eighties, like myself, *got by*. Our parents taught us to keep our heads down and work hard. This idea of meritocracy was very prominent in migrant families at the time. It was partly aspirational — they wanted us to succeed — but it was also safeguarding — they hoped that assimilation into a capitalist workforce would keep us safe from the racism and violence out there.'

Ola went to primary and secondary school in England, and then went back to her home country to study at university. 'It wasn't until I returned to Nigeria that I realised how colonial the British education system is, how many different types of knowledge were intentionally omitted. It made me wonder what we could have learnt of ourselves if these truths weren't hidden.' I ask her what it was like returning to England after university, and she tells me how she got rejected from almost every job she applied for. 'There was an understanding in our communities that certain jobs were not available to Black people no matter how educated we were. The jobs we could get were racist as hell. We'd played by their rules and still couldn't win.'

We discuss how under a capitalist system we're told education is for the young. It prepares us for the labour market, where we are made to spend our healthiest years, and tells us that we will be rewarded with rest upon retirement. The reality is that ageing is rarely restful for those without economic privilege. Though it has continued to rise gradually over the past decade, seventy-one is now being proposed as the new age of retirement in the UK. This, the National Pensioners Convention says, 'will condemn millions of middle-aged people to misery',[4] as was proven in previous years, when the state pension age was raised from sixty-five to sixty-six, and the absolute poverty rate increased by 14 per cent. Where single people, those with fewer educational qualifications and those in rented accommodation were concerned, poverty rates almost doubled.[5]

Despite burnout amid precarity and insecurity being an increasingly common outcome, young people are offered no alternative for their education other than to study hard and work harder. In his book *The Pedagogy of the Oppressed*, Brazilian educator and philosopher Paulo Freire describes the prevailing way we teach and learn in the West as nothing more than a banking system. Education, he observes, has become an act of depositing, in which the teacher is the depositor and the students are the depositories, expected to obediently receive, memorise and regurgitate for the purpose of, for example, exams. This method of banking requires a teacher–student dynamic that reinforces hierarchies of oppression. 'The teacher teaches and the students are taught; the teacher knows everything and the students know nothing [...] the teacher talks and the students listen – meekly; the teacher disciplines and the students are disciplined,'[6] Freire writes.

This formulaic approach to education does little to nurture the next generation of independent thinkers and mobilised doers, instead churning out generation after generation of obedient labourers within a meritocratic capitalist workforce. The academisation of schools has only amplified this. Academies, where a trust or business oversees a series of former state schools, can be understood as the privatisation of education, where young people's socialisation is sacrificed for profit and gain. When high grades and good attendance equals more funding, academies are preoccupied by nothing more than attainment – rather than being concerned with the social health and mental wellbeing of their students.

As a result of such institutional neglect, burnout is normalised. With 85 per cent of students experiencing stress and anxiety about their GCSEs during the pandemic,[7] young people are experiencing the mental health impacts of capitalism before they've even left school. 'Burnout is encouraged through a culture of education that enforces conformity and the idea that our time does not belong to us,' says Aiyana Goodfellow. At seventeen, Aiyana is, among many other endeavours, the founder of Neuromancers, an abolitionist community organisation by and for Black, queer, neurodivergent communities, and co-founder of The Anima Print, a radical Black-led micro-publisher giving a platform to marginalised writers.

Counting on their fingers, Aiyana offers examples of how burnout manifests within education. They relay how young people are expected to prioritise work over their wellbeing, staying up late to revise in order to achieve arbitrary goals such as specific exam grades. Through awards ceremonies and gifted-and-talented programmes, students are praised for overworking, while those who don't are punished through detentions or exclusions and labelled 'bad kids'. Homework trains us to accept unpaid overtime, and uniform encourages conformity. 'Teachers used to tell us to wear our uniform properly on the way to and from school because we're "representing the school",' Aiyana tells me. 'These are all subtle submissions. They teach us that, even when we're not working, our time is not ours.'

'The school system is an extension of the prison industrial complex and is a manifestation of capitalism,' Aiyana continues. 'When child labour laws were introduced, they had to find a place for children to go while their parents work, and schools presented an opportunity to train future generations of workers. So for young people to be liberated from school, we need to abolish capitalism as a whole. Without that abolition of capitalism, there is no youth liberation.'

Education as Transgression

Paulo Freire's pedagogy influenced numerous people's practices, including that of bell hooks. In *Teaching to Transgress*, she talks of growing up among the traumas of her home life and how social theory became a haven for her during this time.

'I found a place of sanctuary in "theorising", in making sense out of what was happening. I found a place where I could imagine possible futures, a place where life could be lived differently. This "lived" experience of critical thinking, of reflection and analysis, became a place where I worked at explaining the hurt and making it go away. Fundamentally, I learned from this experience that theory could be a healing place.'[8]

This mirrors my own experience. Studious and well behaved, I dutifully attended school despite feeling consumed by a viscerally embodied chaos. Though my secondary school was considered one of the worst in Doncaster – and, more recently, made headlines for issuing the highest number of exclusions in the country[9] – at the time it was one of the only, if not the only, schools in the area that offered Sociology as an option from GCSE level. Sociology evidenced that I wasn't crazy, actually. Miss Firth nurtured in me the skill of critical thinking, of laying flat the world around me and mapping the origins of my traumas. It eased the guilt and self-blame I carried, and gave me the language to articulate what was being done to me, to all of us – the fault lay in a carefully constructed system of power and control. Miss Firth's classroom was a safe haven away from the conformity and control of mainstream education. In it, her students were encouraged to challenge the status quo and think critically, and it was here I found a socio-political grounding and theoretical clarity. The seeds of a budding radical were sown.

In an anti-intellectual society where critical thinking is discouraged, hooks recognised theory as the practice of freedom. This, she says, is why it's so important that our liberation struggles continue to centre theory in their practice. 'We must actively work to call attention to the importance of *creating* a theory that can advance renewed feminist movements,' she writes.[10]

Both hooks and Freire emphasise the importance of nurturing a progressive, holistic framework that ensures wellbeing is centred in a learning that transcends age or hierarchy. hooks introduces us to the concept of 'engaged pedagogy', where a teacher's role is to share in the intellectual and spiritual growth of the students, as well as their own. A 'progressive, holistic education, engaged pedagogy is more demanding than conventional critical or feminist pedagogy. For, unlike these two teaching practices, it emphasises wellbeing. That means that teachers must be actively committed to a process of self-actualisation that promotes their own wellbeing if they are to teach in a manner that empowers students.'[11]

Likewise, the 'pedagogy of the oppressed', Freire proposes, is a task for radicals. For people engaged in the fight for their own liberation, this political education and praxis is 'a pedagogy which must be forged with, not for, the oppressed in the incessant struggle to regain their humanity.'[12] Who knows what curriculum we would curate for ourselves if presented with the boundless opportunity to do so. A syllabus that considers Black literature worthy of study, sure, but perhaps also something more profound. A hunger to uncover the familial and ancestral lineages, to learn cultural and land-based practices, to become knowledgeable in the histories of political movements, to explore alternative economies, or to experiment with creative and embodied forms of healing are but a few of my own yearnings. As Freire quotes psychoanalyst and social philosopher Erich Fromm: 'Freedom to create and to construct, to wonder and to venture. Such freedom requires that the individual be active and responsible, not a slave or a well-fed cog in the machine.'[13]

Education as Decolonial Delinquency

In recent years 'Decolonise Education' and, similarly, 'Decolonise the Curriculum' have become two frequent calls to action, drawing attention to the oppressive implications of academia. In her book *Sacred Instructions*, Native American attorney and activist Sherri Mitchell describes the colonial education agenda as one which diminished the worth in all that held meaning for indigenous communities. Suppressing any ideas that may encourage creative, cultural and critical thinking 'kept us fragmented and compartmentalised, and prevented us from reaching our full potential,' she writes.[14]

Mitchell talks of how in indigenous communities elders are recognised as being the guides that empower our relationship with our inner teachers: 'In our bodies, we carry the blood of our ancestors and the seeds of the future generations [...] When we contemplate the vastness of the interwoven network that we are tied to, our individual threads of life seem far less fragile. We are strengthened by who we come from and inspired by those who will follow.'[15]

When I ask Ola about the value of intergenerational organising, she agrees. 'We all have wisdoms to pass on to each other, so centring elders in the movement is an act of care and ensures they are supported in their ageing. It also means that present movements can learn from and build upon the legacies of the past.' Ola offers a weaving metaphor to emphasise the importance of an ancestral pedagogy. 'The racial justice movement today is intricately woven with resistance throughout the ages,' she tells me. 'They evolve and adapt to the issues of time and place, but the thread that connects us is our greatest weapon.'

Considering this in relation to the multi-generational lessons we can learn around burnout, Ola pauses. 'It feels like an interesting dichotomy: previous generations in the UK were burning out due to being subjected to more overt policing and structural insecurity, plus the pressures of first-generation integration. But it could be argued that they built stronger communities and more radical politics as a result. Meanwhile, younger generations are contending with their place as second- or third-generation movement builders. They've also lived with recession after recession and must navigate burnout through the additional prisms of social media and cancel culture for example – our movements weren't perfect, but at least they didn't have *that* to worry about!' She chuckles, before continuing: 'And yet our youth are refusing to be broken by this work. They're finding ways to make this struggle enjoyable and restful, and I'm excited to see how this important message impacts future revolutionaries.'

In considering how we are to nurture the radical potential of our youth, Mitchell recommends that the pathway out of a colonial, capitalist framework is through educational sovereignty. In contrast to a linear model designed to garner dependency through extraction and erasure, an indigenous approach is formed around concentric circles that offer self-determination as an act of 'civil disobedience'. This circular model encompasses all aspects of the child's being – spiritual, individual, familial, communal, global, universal – and 'determines not only who they will become, but who we become as a society', Mitchell writes.[16] Like hooks, she recognises that as those still connected to their inner teacher, who have not yet succumbed to the lures of capitalism, it is young people who should be guiding us. 'We view our children as our teachers, acknowledging that they have as much to show us about the world as we have to show them.'

Speaking with Aiyana, the truth in this becomes abundantly clear. Much of Aiyana's work presently focuses around anti-ageism and youth liberation, and from this they have coined the term 'delinquency' to describe a philosophy of reclaiming how 'misbehaviour' and 'disobedience' are used as a tool to suppress rebellion in young people and, therefore, society. 'Children are seen as inherently irresponsible, and this is reinforced with the opportunity to be responsible taken away from us. All decisions are made for us by adults, or by the state, not by consent. In any other social scenario we would recognise this as oppression, yet we don't consider young people as being in need of freedom,' Aiyana reasons.

In a context where young people have always been at the forefront of rebellion, embracing our delinquency is for everyone. 'What's great is that anybody can be a delinquent. You don't have to be a young person, and you don't have to be someone who was written off as "bad", you just have to be committed to misbehaviour in the name of youth liberation, all liberation,' Aiyana continues, 'I think more of us would like to do that than we might like to admit, because we all have childishness within us – many of us have just repressed it.'

By centring young people as an oppressed group, Aiyana describes delinquency as answering the question of how we can be freer individuals and freer communities. 'When space is held for us to communicate what we want and what we need, it will be these rebellious, imaginative, playful, unrestricted visions that will transform society,'

Aiyana says. I ask them if they can offer examples of what delinquency could look like in practice, and Aiyana smiles. 'Delinquency can look like playful resistance. It can look like restful resistance. It can look like violent resistance,' they explain. 'As an ethics to live by or a structured model of organising for youth liberation, delinquency can look like finding ways to support the children and the parents in your community. Asking, how can we take care of each other's kids? How can we give young people more autonomy, more rest? How can we ensure marginalised families are not isolated under capitalism? How can we surround young people with more caring, safe elders, who are willing to support us? How can we ensure young people's imagination and playfulness are not erased, and how do we ultimately learn from young people?'

Here we begin to understand that those acts more traditionally understood as 'delinquent' – protest or rioting for example – are not bad simply because a carceral system has defined them as such. We also see that to rest, to heal, to be in community, to create, to retreat into nature, to unlearn and relearn in resistance of a capitalist culture of burnout are acts of delinquency. What hooks, Freire, Mitchell and Aiyana conclude is that there is an anarchic potential of a mind that can think critically and in service of every living thing. The earth, our ancestors, the rebellious child and the inner teacher within all of us are the sources of knowledge and wisdom we should be seeking to uncover. And through a decolonial, delinquent pedagogy we may begin to embody the theory – which so often keeps us in our heads and out of our bodies – that we espouse. That the state is so ferociously intent on suppressing the critical thinking and radical imagination of our youth speaks to the revolutionary potential of a decolonised, embodied education – it is this which we must nurture.

On Radical Anxiety

Under oppressive systems that are designed to make us feel detached, disconnected, alienated and isolated, our wellbeing depends on us practicing connecting to each other and the land even if our initial instincts may be to pull away [...] *Living under capitalism's accelerated, fast pace (which is disconnected from nature's slow and gradual cycle of time), instils in us a baseline level of anxiety and fear* [...] *It is no mark of wellness or health to be profoundly well adjusted to its stimuli.*

— Dr Ayesha Khan[1]

Before the waking dread, the dizzying lightheadedness, the relentless overthinking, the spiralling what-ifs, the twisting, cramping sickness, the worst-case scenarios, the dissociative brain fog, the replaying of events, the dysregulated foot tapping, the perpetually tense shoulders, the woefully bedridden days, the panting, breathless panics and the intrusive thoughts that taunt at night, there was a child. A toddler. A baby. Someone who knew nothing of what it means to be alive under racial capitalism.

Diagnosed with an anxiety-cum-panic disorder before I'd even reached my teens, I don't remember that very earliest version of myself. I don't remember a time that preceded anxiousness. It's for this reason that I found communicating the realities and contradictions of anxiety so difficult. Disassociating yet fixating. Subtly subverting the everyday, yet simultaneously world-shattering. A juggling act, yet an emotional numbing. Frequent to the point of normalcy yet disorientating in its power to surprise. Existential, yet deeply personal. Entirely rational, logical, justifiable, yet somehow also absurd, nonsensical, manic. Is there any wonder we burn out?

In the UK, one in six people are affected by anxiety. That's a lot of people who on any given day feel like they're drowning amid a capitalist expectation to stay afloat. In a piece titled 'Be gentle with yourself', the Nigerian poet Ijeoma Umebinyuo suggests that healing itself will come in waves, but that 'maybe today, the wave hits the rocks'.[2] Through the vignettes which follow, I hope to convey the overlapping currents of anxiety that undulate and swell, that lap upon the harbours of the everyday and crash upon the fragile coastlines of a lifetime. And, as with anger and rage, I propose the earnest breakwaters – embodied, communal, nature-allied – that we can build to protect ourselves from the relentless tides of burnout.

Starting in a comfortable seated position, notice your body's contact with the ground beneath you. As you begin to ground yourself in this position, try to find your midline by directing your attention to your spine, the backbone of your body. Feeling the gravitational pull towards the midline allows your spine to align itself with the centre of your body and the centre of the Earth. Close your eyes. As you enter the world of your inner landscape, pay attention to any anxious thoughts that may bubble up when you're relaxed. This may be a personal anxiety, anxiety about the future, or anxiety about the environment. Just sense where that anxiety shows up in the body. When we identify the embodied location

of the anxiety, we can then initiate ways to feel into it.
Everything in our body is connected.

It's about midday on a Wednesday afternoon, and Kalpana Arias and I sit across from each other on Zoom. Kalpana is the founder of Nowadays on Earth, a social enterprise whose work focuses on nature rights, policy and guerrilla gardening. This is not your average gardening club, however. Nowadays on Earth centres an ecosomatics methodology – a trauma-led, decolonial approach that connects growing practices and ecological consciousness with embodied and creative healing.

Kalpana and I first met a year earlier, in that transitional month of November. As autumn turns to winter I, like so many others, reach an uncomfortable state somewhere between despair and desperation. My propensity for joy seems to be entirely depend-ent on the hours of daylight we receive, having so few feels like a punishment. With the winter nights eclipsing all hope, I spend the evenings searching for moments of light amid the darkness. And I found one in Kalpana's ecosomatics workshop: 'Body as Nature'.

Body as Nature was a sensory experience that offered forest therapy as a way to connect with the more-than-human world, and it took place the day after bonfire night. My partner and I decided to join the online workshop while on a walk along our local woodland trail. We perched on a bench overlooking a duck pond that sits at the foot of shadowy greenhouses, lining the hilled allotments against a moonlit sky. Conjoined by a pair of wired headphones, Kalpana's soothing practice instructed us in one ear, while the conversation between invisible moorhens dominated the other. Residual fireworks erupted into explosive constellations in the distance, and there we bore witness to the colliding of the human and more-than-human. I became entranced with Kalpana's practice that day, and today I'm here to interview her on the ways ecosomatics can support those with climate anxiety. But as with so much of this work, sometimes showing is more powerful than telling. We find ourselves in an impromptu session, with Kalpana giving me a taste of her practice:

> *Pay attention to wherever you feel anxiety in your body. Maybe it's your chest, your stomach, or your head. Take a few breaths here, breathing into the area of your body where you feel anxiety. Then let it travel throughout your body, until it reaches your hands. Imagine you are holding the anxiety in your hands, take another breath, and as you exhale start to open your fingers and let your hands hold the space between them. Let your fists unclench, and your wrists relax a little. When you feel you're not holding so tightly on to your anxiety, you can start to have a conversation with it. What is your anxiety trying to say to you? What voice does it speak in?*

Ecosomatics, Kalpana explains, allows us to go into the fundamental experience of learning how to be. 'We're not taught how to move through the world, in nature, with these bodies that hold different experiences in such complex ways,' she says. When we disassociate from our bodies, and from the anxiety they hold within them, it also becomes impossible for us to have a relationship with the natural world around us. 'Ecosomatics allows you to go into a dialogue between your body and your immediate surroundings so that you can experience the multitude of perspectives that live within. It's a tool of reclamation. Nature rights groups and campaigns often talk about re-commoning the lands, well, through this experiential practice we're also re-commoning our bodies,' she expands.

What I love about Kalpana's approach to embodied practice is the way it offers nature connection, in particular gardening, as both a metaphor for our relationship with the natural world, and a solution to our disconnection from it. Racial capitalism tells us to manage and maintain our emotional gardens, rather than creating a thriving biodiverse relationship with them. Instead of this vision of control, Kalpana tries to see anxiety and burnout as tension points where our body starts to contract, telling us that we need to find a sense of safety. If we listen to them, if we act, she says, there's the opportunity here – as with any garden, as with our world at large – to create a wilder, more reciprocal landscape that allows for healing. When anxiety, hopelessness and despair thrive on our individualised isolation from land, each other and our bodies, the more we feel part of something, the less power it has over us.

As Kalpana says to me at the end of our Zoom conversation, in words that immediately bring a smile to my face: 'Through gardening you witness, intimately, the magic of evolutionary decay and rebirth, and suddenly the end of things doesn't feel so anxiety inducing. We can see the end of one thing – the end of this capitalist world in which fossil fuel companies are literally creating burnout, for example – as an opportunity for something beautiful.'

Can you start to see this feeling of anxiety as a message from the body that's alerting you to something or trying to convey a narrative to you? Does this change how you might greet this anxiety? With patience, with grace? What do you say back to that anxiety? What do you invite in? And what do you let go? Slowly, intentionally, move your hands to the ground and experience the body and Earth as one as you feel the ground hold these anxieties for you. Breathe into your hands, and into the ground – this is the dialogue between your body and land.

~◯

It's the end of summer 2023 and it's not just us humans that are burning out. Our planet is also on fire, figuratively and literally. Between the months of July and September, wildfires ravished parts of Europe, Asia, North Africa and North America. In the first week of September alone, Greece, Turkey, Libya, Brazil, Hong Kong, Shanghai and Spain all experienced severe floods. Morocco experienced its worst earthquake in forty years, and the USA set a new record for climate disasters following hurricanes that devastated Florida. The UK government has just approved the Rosebank Oil Field, the biggest undeveloped oil field in the British North Sea, which will release more emissions than 700 million people in the so-called Global South. And the war against the peoples of the Middle East is yet to begin, which will not only claim thousands upon thousands of lives but will also produce more planet-warming gases in the first few months than twenty climate-vulnerable nations do in a year.

These disasters aren't natural. Rather, they are the product of colonial legacies which led to the destruction of ecosystems and communities through extraction. Communities of colour are disproportionately impacted by the real-time impacts of climate and humanitarian crises, and of the increasingly fascist states that sanction the environmental plundering of people and the planet. Lives, destroyed. Land, decimated. Communities, displaced. The Stockholm Resilience Centre recently released a detailed map of the nine planetary boundaries held by Earth, showing how climate change is affecting each of them. These boundaries, which signify the planet's limitations, include: climate change, novel entities, stratospheric ozone depletion, atmospheric aerosol loading, ocean acidification, landsystem change, biogeochemical flows, freshwater change and biosphere integrity. Of these nine boundaries, six of them have been crossed significantly, the report says.

Well that's not good, I mutter to myself, before turning my phone face down on the coffee table and reaching for an Amazon remote control, created by a guy in the wealthiest 1 per cent of people on this burning planet. I used to be something of a reality TV snob, internally judging those who chose to spend their time watching fame-hungry ants scurry around on screen. At some point during one of the lockdowns, however, I succumbed, welcoming the numbness it offers. I reasoned that the sociologist in me could find fascination in the social experiment of it all. I was partially correct. But mostly, I'm just relieved by the distraction, and allow it to make me a bystander in the impending environmental collapse. Anything to avoid thinking too hard, feeling too hard, about the latest disaster.

The writer and climate activist Tori Tsui has written that 'eco-anxiety is a rational, natural and adaptive response to truly irrational and unnatural circumstances such as climate change'[3] and, given that I'm riddled with it, I find this reassuring. It aligns with my own work around validating and understanding emotional responses to a trauma. And that is what the climate crisis is, after all: incremental traumas that we witness and experience in differing degrees of powerlessness and impact. The ways the psychological toll of climate uncertainty manifests as avoidance – reality TV and all – bears many similarities to the freeze and fawn trauma responses that I'm well versed in. An avoidance of abject worry, fear, hopelessness and despair, though they're felt all the same. It's defined by a sense of powerlessness, a lack of control. And, historically, when I have had my agency and control removed from me, I simply submit. That's what I'm doing now, resigned to my fate, on my pink velvet sofa in front of the TV screen. Submitting.

Yet as I doomscroll through Instagram, a post made by Steve Misati, a Kenyan climate activist working with the youth-led organisation The Resilience Project, tells me that inertia doesn't have to paralyse us. Eco-anxiety embodies a multitude of emotions: dread, anger, numbness, fear, shame, powerlessness, excitement and joy, but 'by acknowledging our concerns, adopting coping strategies, and taking meaningful action, we can transform eco-anxiety into a catalyst for positive change,' he says.[4] And it's in this that I find myself a site of constant contradiction when it comes to climate anxiety, fluctuating between the Jekyll and Hyde states of hopeful movement-builder on the one hand, harnessing imaginative abolitionist and eco-centric frameworks with Peaks of Colour, and, on the other, the anxious-avoidant doomsayer that I become when permitted a moment's silence at home. Exhausting.

Nineteenth-century terraced houses in Sheffield aren't made for the climates of the present day. In the winter, central heating is no match for their draughty bones, and in summer . . . well, in summer, it's hot. It's the kind of heat that reminds you that the world is on fire with every bead of sweat you wipe from your brow. With a fan whirring in the background, hopping on a Zoom call with Dominique Palmer is a welcome distraction.

Dominique is a climate justice activist, writer, storyteller and speaker whose work focuses on intersectionality and youth power in climate movement spaces. This is our first-ever meeting, which is surreal given that social media has allowed me to feel so intimately up to date in her work. Dom has just come back from speaking on youth activism at an event alongside Greta Thunberg. She's also recently finished her undergraduate degree in political science and international affairs, been the subject of a Q&A at the Southbank Centre about climate joy and optimism, was front and centre of the Stop Rosebank march, and has just finished touring for a book she co-authored with 2,500 schoolchildren.

I'm grateful that Dom's found time to speak with me amid such a busy schedule. She says it's come at a time where she's recognising in herself a need for rest. She knows the warning signs, she tells me, and anxiety is one of them. 'Eco-anxiety, for me, comes in waves. When I'm in this work, I wake up and confront the climate crisis every day, so the emotions don't always hit me. But eventually it adds up to the point where a wave of anxiety crashes.' Like a lot of us, the news is often what instigates this, but in Dom's work, anxiety also follows when she attends mainstream climate events. By way of example she offers the United Nations Climate Change Conferences (the COP meetings), from which she returned recently. 'So much of my anxiety comes from spending time with those in power who continue to make the decisions that put us further into climate breakdown,' she expands. 'Climate anxiety isn't our personal fault or failure, it's a result of the systems that we exist in that have created this condition.'

Another, perhaps surprising, trigger for Dominique is climate doomism – the mistaken belief that we're past the point of no return and that mankind is likely to become extinct: 'Climate doomism is something that incredibly frustrates me because it comes from inactivity. In a weird way it can actually give me more climate anxiety. Not because I believe that we're too late to change anything – the science tells us that we do have time – but because

I know we need to mobilise more people and this message of hopelessness actually turns people away.'

Contrastingly, Dom tells me of the number of people within the environmental movement who are burning out due to eco-anxiety, the very thing that brought them to these spaces in the first place. She sighs, then adds, 'I'm now noticing that because a lot more young people are engaging with this work through fear, they then approach the work with urgency. It pushes this "ends justify the means" approach to organising, meaning that collective care and justice are actually ignored to the extent that climate actions can be really dangerous. We talk about sustainable futures, but when we're not resourced and when our wellbeing isn't centred, our present movements become unsustainable.'

We discuss how, when channelled in this way, our anxiety can become a means of our own destruction, making people into collateral damage in a cycle of crisis. As Dominique underlines: '*How* we do the work is just as important as *what* we do.' What Dom and I are more interested in, then, is how our anxiety can become a tool of imagination and transformation rather than something grinding us down, and not only in environmental spaces. I ask her how she approaches this in her work. 'Being anxious about something shows you care. It shows how much love and passion you have about the thing you want to protect,' she considers. 'That in itself can be the start of transformation. I had my big turning point when I went to COP25 in 2019. I put so much energy into it, and came out feeling completely shaken, because I was grappling with a system that really isn't fit for purpose. This may have been the first time I experienced burnout, that deep anxiety.'

In the wake of this, Dominique took a break and started looking for ways of working that didn't feel so awful, that felt *good*. 'You know, this work can be very serious,' she tells me, 'but I've always been that person that seeks joy, especially childlike joy, playfulness, and yet here I was in a climate space that wasn't bringing me anything like joy.' Dom initially started making time for joyful activities as a way to balance the stresses of climate spaces. Eventually, however, the two began to merge. 'Climate Live, for example, came from an idea my friend had where we brought people together to sing, but also to engage, empower and educate. I'd always loved singing and theatre. Music has a way of touching people, emoting people.' It's this sense of joyful practice that she's kind enough to recognise in Peaks of Colour too. Nature brings out a kind of playfulness and celebration in community. Dom reflects, 'I really do feel like I've been on a big journey of something I call climate joy, of trying to cultivate joy in a crisis, which can be difficult, but it's very, very possible.' I note the strength of the word 'possible' and its ability to quell the most powerful waves of anxiety. And as I witness Dom speak about this, her body lifts with a restless energy, her face alight with smiles. The embodied evidence of all that is possible.

On this day, there are just two of us, Hafsah and me. It's a grey afternoon in January, drizzly and overcast, and though a large floor lamp creates a cosy atmosphere, the low clouds darken Hafsah's dining room. It matches my mood. I am tense. Present yet disengaged. As I'm faced with the seemingly infinite number of tasks on Peaks of Colour's to-do list, there is little sense of joy and possibility here right now. I feel decidedly overwhelmed. Hafsah has offered to help me get these thoughts out of my head — where they're succeeding in completely consuming me in a storm of anxiety — and onto paper, in an ordered, aesthetically pleasing fashion.

I first met Hafsah when she joined a Peaks of Colour walk, and we bonded quite quickly over the ability to approach the same vision from two completely different yet complementary angles. Strategy and imagination aligned. Today I need her focus, her Mary Poppins-like bag of exercises and skill for drawing out the best in people. That and her array of sticky notes, obnoxiously colourful amid the grey hues of my mood and the weather.

Throughout the morning she asks me questions, writing on and reordering the sticky notes with confidence. Her ability to understand me, to translate my jumbled-up thoughts into a coherent action, is comforting, and I feel myself relaxing into the process. Eventually she puts down her pen, standing up and peering over her work, hands on hips. 'Okay, I think we're done,' she says confidently. Before us lies a multicoloured road map for the year ahead. Under each monthly heading sits a rainbow of sticky notes, a breakdown of all the practical, organisational things that need to be done, month by month, in order for Peaks of Colour to actualise a transformative vision.

It was clear and concise. Challenging, yet not overly ambitious. Doable. And yet while the road map made Hafsah feel prepared, it was making me feel panicked. A familiar churning began to rise in the pit of my stomach, followed by a light-headedness and a bubbling nausea. The session was meant to make us feel excited for the months ahead, yet I was consumed with this foreboding dread. Feeling embarrassed, and guilty for having wasted Hafsah's time, I excused myself and quickly made a dash for the toilet. This scenario used to be painfully frequent, where a situation would make me feel either so anxious or unsafe or triggered that I'd find myself rushing to the loo numerous times in one day, rapidly losing weight alongside all sense of reality.

The gut contains 500 million neurons, which are connected to the brain through the nervous system. It also contains neurotransmitters (chemicals, such as serotonin, which are produced by the brain and control feelings and emotions), alongside microbes that are stored or produced in the gut. The nervous system is recognised to be an intricate network of nerves and cells that line the gastrointestinal tract and connect the gut to the brain. The vagus nerve is one such intra-connector, assisting digestion and telling the body how to behave. In Ayurvedic medicine, the gut is considered the 'second brain' for this reason. And this physical and biochemical communication is known as the gut–mind connection. In this reciprocal relationship, stress has been found to inhibit the signals sent through the vagus nerve, causing gastrointestinal, mental health and cognitive problems. An unhealthy or dysregulated gut can affect brain health, but, conversely, mental health conditions like anxiety can also impact the gut, causing, as I call them, nervous poos.

Back in Hafsah's home, this was a clear warning sign that something wasn't right. I peeled myself off the cold tiles of the bathroom floor, which I'd been using to ground myself, and gradually re-emerged into the dining room. It didn't seem an option to not be honest in this moment. To be anything other than vulnerable, to not show up, flaws and all, felt disrespectful to Hafsah and to the work, so I told her about my anxious bowels. 'I know that this is my body telling me that something doesn't feel right about this, but I can't put my finger on exactly what,' I said.

Grateful for Hafsah's patience, I watched as she moved around some of the sticky notes, looked for my reaction and tried again. Eventually I gasped. 'This! This feels good!' The nervous churning in my tummy subsided as quickly as it had erupted, and I felt like the rain cloud that was following me around had lifted, passed across my chest, then moved on.

We peered over the pages that lay before us – a new road map, which signalled a considerably different journey to the ones either of us had envisioned. January, February, March, April, May: blank pages. I started to laugh, feeling stupid and slightly confused by my ability to make such a glaring omission first time around. 'The book!' In all our plotting and planning, we had forgotten that Peaks of Colour remains just a small part of our respective works. I had just signed this very book deal a few months before, and with a quick turnaround deadline looming, we couldn't maintain a business-as-usual approach to Peaks of Colour, because the upcoming year would be anything but usual. Clearing our diary in order to allow me enough space and time to write had to be a priority. My body, my gut, had remembered this even when my brain had not, and there was a lesson in this. What once could have felt like a huge decision and upheaval – to pause the monthly walks for the rest of the year – in fact gave us a comforting satisfaction.

It was then that we vowed to include 'Embodied Organising' as a core principle of Peaks of Colour's practice. Gone are the days of anxiety being an unwritten requirement of our job description. Instead, we express a commitment to listening to our bodies so that we can move through only what feels good. It is an exciting thought, to consider the different directions your work could take if you dismissed arbitrary obligations and embraced only positive experiences. What if tasks could be assigned by what felt comfortable and exciting for each person, as opposed to a list of roles on a job description? What if when something didn't feel right in a particular moment – maybe because we're menstruating or feeling under the weather – we simply came back to it at a time when it did? What if when faced with a task that was simply unavoidable, something that sits outside our comfort zones, we worked in an embodied way to ensure that we made it as cushioned as possible – taking that work outside, increasing the snacks, including more people, making movement a part of the process?

Learning to listen to our bodies, beginning to understand what they are telling us, is only the starting point of an embodied practice. Doing so allows us to begin to differentiate between what doesn't feel good because it's triggering old wounds that need attending to, and what doesn't feel good because it's a symptom of capitalism, for which alternatives need to be found. It's common for us to doubt and question ourselves, to feel overwhelmed by an anxiety born out of all we feel we must do and must be, but this place of hypervigilance, scarcity and trauma is no place from which to build a movement. The more we strengthen this muscle of building embodied skills, the more we deepen our trust in ourselves and each other. The more we increase our resilience and capacity for what feels good, the more *doing* this work becomes, in and of itself, an expansive opportunity for transformation.

How does it feel to be as free as a bird? This is the question we sought to answer during 'Embodying Liberatory Freedoms', the second walkshop in a series with the Right to Roam campaign. As we idled along the Rivelin Valley Trail, a nature trail which takes walkers from the Sheffield suburbs into the Peak District, ornithologist and Right to Roam campaigner Nadia Shaikh led us in a birdwatching and nature meditation walkshop.

On this journey, which took place during Refugee Week, and as part of the Migration Matters Festival, we grappled with binoculars, attuning our bird identification techniques through song as well as sight, considering the contradictions projected on the human and the more-than-human. The migration of birds, for example, has long been celebrated. Year after year, season after season, the arrival of swifts and swallows from their winter homes elicits rejoicing and jubilation. It's anticipated. The arrival of refugees and asylum seekers, however, persecuted and destitute, evokes repugnant hostility. Despite our movement being incited by the same conditions as those birds – climate displacement, unrest, resources, survival – for people of colour, our migration is often met with suspicion at the borders we humans have constructed.

There's a sadness in recognising that as racialised communities, we, and the ancestors who came before us, are well versed in understanding why the caged bird sings but are yet to know the same freedoms as a redwing or a chiffchaff. A life free from restrictions, from scrutiny, from policing, from struggle, from heartache and the hypervigilance, tension, stress, and the anxiety it causes within us. *What would it be like to exist in our bodies safely?* we asked.

In the second half of the walkshop, we were introduced to the ways somatics could be a political practice by movement artist, performer and facilitator Sym Stellium. As a welcome rain shower permeated the heat of a sweltering June afternoon, Sym led us in movement and visualisation exercises, where we practised taking up space in the grounds of a private land-cum-community centre, filling it in ways that felt instinctive and natural.

As part of this, Sym challenged us to focus on two parts of our bodies: firstly, where we felt the most tension; secondly, where we felt the most release. 'How does this part of our body feel'? Sym asked. 'What message is it trying to convey to us? If we were to move through that part of the body, in what ways would it guide us? Contort us? Lead us into new positions and ways of being?'

I started noticing a prickling, stabbing sensation, small but sharp, along the hairline at the nape of my neck. My body jolted with every shock of pain. A few months previously I had been incapacitated by a trapped nerve in the back of my neck. I'd woken up one morning unable to move and, despite having recovered gradually, was still experiencing residual aches. So feeling pain here didn't surprise me. The depths of realisation that emerged from Sym's prompts, however, certainly did. *What message could this sensation be trying to convey?* With each shock came an image: a snapshot of a man hanging from a door frame with a rope around his neck. Though I'd never seen my grandad in the place in which he took his own life, my rampant childhood imagination had pictured it many times. A self-inflicted torture that would induce my earliest panic attacks. Another electric shock along my hairline jolted me from the projected memory to a present state of understanding. These emotional wounds not only plant seeds of anxiety within us; when left unattended, they also manifest in the physical. Perhaps this seemingly unrelated trapped nerve was a message, a reminder of what remains unaddressed, and an assurance that now is the time to do so. With Sym's direction I gave my neck gentle stretches and noticed how, as I instinctively elongated it, it led the way, tilting my head back so that my face was lifted towards the sky. A hopeful, rooting action.

Following the second prompt to move through what felt good, the part of the body that really spoke to me was the balls of my feet. What I noticed, however, was that the soles of my feet felt hot. A pulsating, aching heat that throbbed in my walking boots. I felt compelled to remove them and sooth my feet on the cool, damp grass. The more I paid attention to this heat, the more the sensation started to travel, up through my toes, to my ankles, the backs of my calves, thighs, lower back, spine, shoulders, neck and temple, until my whole body began to tingle. It wasn't uncomfortable. Rather, it felt like the immediate release after a massage. *I must look after my feet*, I thought. *They transport me through this healing journey.*

When it came to sharing what arose for us in the session, I found I wasn't the only person who had been drawn to their neck that day. One person reflected how conscious they were that their neck was trapped between their head and body, like an in-between land, a liminal space that often gets neglected. Others felt called to examine their relationship with the inner workings of their neck, their throat and tongue. People reflected on the ways they're instrumental as a tool of oral traditions, or how it could represent the holding of your tongue – an enforced silence. 'For me, it was the front of my neck,' one person said. 'It didn't make much sense to me at first, then I thought of the two veins that always appeared in my mum's neck when she was stressed. That's how we knew she was angry or anxious.' A relatable chorus of 'mmm's sounded in solidarity. 'It made me think of all the tension that has been built up over generations, that appears in bloodstreams. All the tension from staying silent instead of expressing the feelings, because for whatever reason, we know we can't.' Ancestral trauma was something that came up regularly.

With Sym's guidance, we were able to feel at peace, present and rooted in place rather than at the unruly behest of our emotions. They remind us that the goal of healing isn't to be always regulated, but to move through dysregulation with greater ease, and so, even when a bee buzzes past our ear, we remain still and in connection with it. Even when the rain falls on our faces, we remain present within it. Even when the wind howls through the leaves of the trees, we embrace the loud soundscape of nature. Any anxieties about the past or future had no place here. What stood out to me that day was how the freedom we felt as we returned from the walkshop had been contingent on us feeling through the pain in our bodies. This wasn't about denying our anxieties or stresses but identifying the sites of transformation that needed our attention. Exploring embodied responses to liberations/oppressions and freedoms/unfreedoms repositioned our bodies not as mere recipients of systemic harms but as maps. And we were the cartographers, journeying through the peaks and valleys of anxiety, stress, togetherness and joy, until we returned home to ourselves.

We moved a lot when I was a child. The house we stayed in the longest, however, sits on a quiet row of council houses in an area of Doncaster that's considered to be 'rough as fuck'. Regardless, this street housed me, my grandparents and three of my oldest friends. From our front doors we would follow an alleyway alongside the allotments, go through the park and around the back of the play area. Hidden next to the rowing club sat the entrance to the River Don, and here we would while away many a weekend, playing along its banks.

This river mapped much of my childhood. With my grandparents, this landscape was experienced as a jungle in which to be played in. Here I was introduced to ivy, hawthorn, elm, yew, beech, chestnut, sycamore, buckthorn, pine and poplar – in feeling if not yet by name. My friends and I, after calling for each other one by one, would embark on a multitude of adventures, exploring the many routes it offered. In winter we would cross the viaduct and continue along the dusty bike track until we reached the grounds of Cusworth Hall, whose hills were the perfect landscape for sledging in the snow. At other times we would go under the bridge, following the river, then through woodlands that lifted us high above the water to where sunlight streamed over a tapestry of farmland. Journeying on, past the fragrant wild garlic that grows in late spring, at the weir which marks the entrance to a nature reserve, we'd patiently wait to see the resident heron announce itself among the bulrushes. To continue further would see us joining the Trans Pennine Trail, a thirty-mile expedition that follows the River Don to Sheffield, which we always vowed we'd do one day.

As a teenager who felt consumed with emotions, I would return here alone in search of isolation and escape. This riverside became a hideaway where I was able to voice or make sense of all the anxieties of an abusive relationship that I bottled up so efficiently. It was in the intimacies of these moments that I would become acclimated to a specific scent, one which I came to associate with patience and trust in the process, helping me to believe that even the most painful of days, the most breathless of panic attacks, the most sinister of intrusive thoughts, can pass. It's the sickly sweet earthiness of Himalayan balsam. A sunset of colour: thick red-orange stems supporting clusters of dainty helmet-shaped flowers in hues of purple and pink, towering above. They still make me feel at home.

Also known as *Impatiens glandulifera*, Himalayan balsam can grow to heights of seven feet. Along the River Don it eclipses the riverbank on its right and suffocates the sounds of the train tracks to the left. For me, wading through the velvety leaves has always signified a sense of solitude. That it is now safe to let the overwhelming emotions escape me. Despite the route being a public footpath, used regularly by locals, on this walk it could be hours before your path crossed with another person. This presented ample time for self-regulation, and among the *Impatiens* I came to understand the magic of being able to root into relationship with a place. Encountering a passer-by, a dog walker, fisherman or cyclist, however, would elicit a visceral reaction. It felt like they were trespassing, not on the land — after all, it wasn't mine to keep — but on the secrets and shame I had laid to rest there.

It was during one such emotion-fuelled expedition that I was first introduced to land justice. I had come across two older white men who were hacking away at the Himalayan balsam with shears. I felt an overwhelming powerlessness, that the one lifeline I could rely on was being taken from me. I was just as surprised at my bravery as they were when I began shouting at them. But it wasn't long before their smirks dismissed the teenager who had appeared from nowhere, and I fled to the sounds of metallic destruction. Though this was not why the men were felling it (the path was too overgrown for their dogs to walk through, they told me), I have since learned that the Himalayan balsam is considered an invasive species. Each plant can produce up to 800 seeds and — much like intrusive thoughts — these are dispersed widely as the ripe pods project them up to seven metres away. The plant then grows rapidly and spreads quickly — much like an anxiety attack — smothering other vegetation as it goes. Himalayan balsam flowers throughout spring, summer and autumn, then — much like my ability to remain optimistic during a depressive episode — it begins to die in winter.

When I revisit my childhood sanctuary after many grief-stricken years, it's autumn. A crunching carpet of conker shells leads me into a tunnel of foliage, which begins to congeal into a squelching footpath — there's been a period of heavy rain — and I have to take care to avoid slipping into the mud. Soon the enclosed passage opens up, and I'm faced by the stillness of the river on my right. It's a wide body of water, known for its filth, yet the cows in the field opposite are lapping at its brown, foamy edges. It takes me a moment to recognise, then appreciate, how unchanged this landscape is. How I am still able to find the breath that escapes me during anxious moments, and how little I understood my dependency upon this place in my youth. The relationships I once shared here may now be unrecognisable, but my other friends, the *Impatiens*, resilient and trustworthy, turn to greet me. It feels apt that I should continue to find home and understanding amid such an ecologically resilient species, I realise. They continue to survive and endure, and so have I. And nature reminds me, once again, that our anxieties bring an awareness to the injustices we need to attend to, and point us in the direction of freedom.

On Radical Abundance

Maybe 'the point' isn't to live more, in the literal sense of a
longer or more productive life, but rather, to be more alive
in any given moment – a movement outward and across,
rather than shooting forward on a narrow, lonely track.
                            – Jenny Odell[1]

I t's an unseasonably rainy day in July, and I find myself once again on the phone to Universal Credit. Placed on hold for the third time in twenty minutes, I sit, mindlessly scrolling Twitter. I'm trying to quell the anxiety attacks that arise when navigating the hostility of statutory services in order to have my basic needs met. *#KingCharles* is trending, and I find my thumb obediently reaching for whatever infuriating news story is about to break. My cheeks flush with instant regret as I read the headline: 'King Charles to receive huge pay rise'.[2] In 2025, the *Guardian* piece stated, King Charles's annual income will increase from £86 million to £125 million, due to government plans to boost public funding of the monarchy by 45 per cent. This story came less than a week after news broke that if Labour were to win the next general election, they would not scrap the two-child benefit cap: Keir Starmer (since labelled 'Sir Kid Starver' by the furious) 'defends decision',[3] said the paper. When the alternative would be to lift 270,000 households with children out of poverty, this decision can only be described as systemic inhumanity. The abundance of the haves rubbed in the faces of the have-nots.

Under racial capitalism, scarcity is certainly an emotion. It feels like a bone-chilling iciness, with almost 5,000 preventable deaths caused by the impact of cold homes during each British winter.[4] It feels like stomach-rumbling hunger, with one in five UK households skipping meals, going hungry or not eating for a whole day amid gross food insecurity. It feels like despair and dependency, with 30 per cent of jobseekers finding they're unable to sustain the cost of living on their meagre salaries.[5] It feels like a lack of home, shelter and security, with a 29 per cent rise in first-time rough sleepers since the rise in inflation led to the cost-of-living crisis.[6] It's a feeling of running on empty, of living in a constant state of *just* about surviving (never mind thriving), of our nervous systems being forever in crisis mode while meeting our basic needs becomes increasingly unattainable. This overbearing sense of lack is inextricable from our experiences of burnout.

When we speak of abundance, therefore, it is in direct response to this perverse scarcity. It's not about having more than we need – there are plenty of people already operating from that space (*gives bombastic side eye to King Charles and the more than 2,800 millionaires, not to mention the fifty or so billionaires, in our one small country*). Abundance, when discussed within social justice spaces, is simply advocating for an equitable distribution of wealth and resources without over-extracting from the resource itself. Having safe homes to return to, healthy food to feed our families, some expendable income to save for our future or treat ourselves, because why not? Having regular time and space away from work in accessible landscapes where we can rest and recuperate – essential, as we've seen in the first few chapters, to the embodied ways we connect with our exhaustion, grief, rage and anxiety. Having a life that is not defined by the productivity of our labour and which nourishes relationships that nurture and sustain us shouldn't be too much to ask. When our basic needs are denied, however, burnout is not a possibility — it's a certainty.

This exploration of radical abundance is the first of four chapters focusing on 'positive' emotions through which we might resist burnout. Taking a different approach to those chapters and emotions we've explored so far, what you'll find here are a series of conversations held with five organisers whose work addresses what it means to be resourced — that is, to have everything we need to survive and thrive so that we can continue doing the work of liberating ourselves from burnout, oppression and scarcity in its many forms.

The honesty and vulnerability, the dark humour and the banter, the ways in which ideas, excitements and enthusiasms bounce off each other, how we challenge each other to think and feel into our own becoming — these are all depicted in these interviews. These conversations are raw, unapologetic examples of how we speak with each other when in movement together, so there felt little need for me to translate or contextualise. These organisers are the theory and the practice personified. In their visions, we can see how an abundant future, in which we are resourced beyond our burnout, is not idealistic, but entirely possible. And so, I let their words speak for themselves.

Abundance as Money:
In Conversation with Seyi Falodun-Liburd

Seyi Falodun-Liburd is the co-director of feminist campaign group Level Up and co-founder of Project Tallawah, an emerging Black Feminist resourcing and community initiative. Together Seyi and I explore the resource at the heart of so many of our experiences of lack — money — and the potential for a landscape of transformative funding for our movements in the long term.

Transformative funding: an expansive model of funding in which funds are distributed to those excluded from mainstream funding and charity regimes. It disrupts and reimagines the dominant power structures within philanthropic spaces.

EM: In what way does our current economy perpetuate burnout among those of us doing movement work?

SFL: So, if abundance is being resourced, then burnout is scarcity. Funders have millions, billions – figures that feel unimaginable to the likes of you and I – yet they fuel scarcity by only funding a handful of organisations, when thousands upon thousands apply. There is this deeply ingrained practice of benevolence in the philanthropy space, and funders drip-feed money because they deem activists as untrustworthy, as incapable of managing their money correctly. But the people who do this work are probably the most financially savvy people that I know, actually. Constantly doing the most with the least. I know funders see this in their reports every time that organisations are over-delivering. We burn out because we're forced to become financial managers, accountants, auditors on top of the work we already do, and yet, there is *still* this lack of trust in these positions.

Which means it's very difficult for movements to do forward-thinking work from a place of scarcity. I'll give an example of long-term strategic thinking: the overturning of Roe v. Wade [which had granted the right to abortion in the USA] was the result of twenty years of campaigning by 'pro-life' – no, *pro-control* – advocates. Twenty years ago, after the Roe v. Wade ruling, they said, 'Ah, we need to start moving.' They had money, they had time, and they were able to connect on their hatred of abortion. But the way we're funded prevents us from doing that forward thinking, that coalition building, that resourcing. If funders are *really* serious about resourcing change, they would be acting on how to ensure a coalition of organisations can be resourced for ten, twenty, thirty years' work.

EM: It's interesting because us being resourced enough to create greater freedoms still feels like a dream, but when fascists want to be resourced enough to restrict our freedoms further, it easily becomes a reality. Peaks of Colour has just been funded for two years, and even though we've been given the most money I've ever seen, in the back of my mind is: 'What do we do after that?' I feel like I'd fallen into the trap I was trying to resist.

SFL: Exactly, and that shouldn't be taking up space in your head. How can you be strategic if you don't have the time and the resources to deepen the work that you're already doing? And then you've gotta create new work to be funded again, instead of continuing what's working.

EM: I'm just thinking, I don't think I've ever come across funding that covers ten years, five years even.

SFL: And it's so frustrating, because during the Black uprisings and the pandemic in 2020, funders were suddenly *very* flexible about how they could do things, how quickly they can send money, about what barriers could be removed. And we're just seeing a regression back into business as usual, rather than an expansion of what was generated at that time.

EM: There's something about urgency within scarcity as well, and who gets to decide what's urgent. The pandemic was, for a time, immediately defined, and rightly so, as urgent – although the Tories had a pathetic way of showing it – but every other social justice issue isn't afforded that level of urgency.

SFL: Urgency, control, dependency, scarcity, they're all interlinked. When Level Up was coming back after the pandemic, we realised that we'd become stuck in this cycle of project funding. Like you said, juggling all these different projects, which meant that people stopped being paid once the project's finished. Very strategically, we were like, we're not doing project funding anymore. Core funding only. Now, there's very few funders who only offer core funding. So that shrinks the pool. We were clear that there's a specific way we want to be funded. Through funders who trust us to do the work. No money is clean, but some money is cleaner than others, so we're picky, and that again shrank the already small pool. Level Up are working towards not existing anymore, and we want funders who support that 'development into degrowth', almost. We're trying to shift things so that survival, and existing in perpetuity, is no longer necessary.

EM: Which brings me to my next question, as I know your work with Project Tallawah is grounded in principles and practices of how we change all of what we've just been discussing. Could you talk me through this?

SFL: Yeah, sure. For Project Tallawah, from the beginning we talked about what the container was going to be. Initially we were an unregistered organisation, then we were hosted by another organisation, then we became a co-op. And I say this because I think that really sets the tone for the amount of granular detail that we go into in order to try and resist this white supremacist system. Language is also really important. We're not funders, we're sharing money.

We're also very clear about who we centre, and who we are doing this work for: African and Caribbean, and global majority heritage women and gender-expansive communities. Growing and building that community is our only intention, alongside ensuring people are resourced to do what they need to do. And I don't just mean meeting the immediate needs, making payroll or paying rent for the building. It's also a question of how we make and resource space to rest, create, make art, connect with each other. Our point of view comes from us being of and within the movement, and not an overseer of the movement. All of us at Project Tallawah hold lots of different capacities and projects in movement spaces, and we bring our experiences to that space. This means we're not interested in following the same format as philanthropic funding, we're all tired of that.

It's interesting, people come with a whole proposal, a budget, and deliverables. And we're like, we understand why you did that, but you don't have to with us. Our approach is that we get to know communities and actually understand what it is they need. I think for a lot of people, it's an uncomfortable experience initially, because we're very conditioned into this capitalist way of how we get money.

EM: Begging, essentially!

SFL: Begging – exactly! You go through that long process of begging.

EM: Normalised begging. Professionalised begging!

SFL: And we're just not interested in that at all. Because a lot of the time when we budget, we make our budgets the smallest they possibly can be, so that they don't think we're asking for too much, then say no. It diminishes your power. A lot of the time we have to push back and say, 'It sounds like you need more.' Our role is to support people to go from that place of survival to a place of dreaming. If our needs are being met, what else?

EM: What's been the responses so far from people you're working with, who have been gifted the ability to imagine and to dream?

SFL: Oh, God, I have goosebumps right now. I get a bit emotional, because it's been two years of trying to create something that only existed in our imagination, so when you're in the room with the communities you shared the money with, it's a lot. But there's also a huge value in the connection that we've all been able to establish. We found so much of our time has just been holding people to share and speak about how they feel doing this work. To *feel* the feelings, because in a lot of spaces there isn't necessarily the permission to do that. There were people in the room who said they hadn't spoken about certain issues in ten years, they hadn't cried about the work in twenty years, but in that space they felt they could, and they did. This really highlighted the value of this work because it was clear that once that immediate need is met, it gives space to just *feel*. For me, it's energising and heartbreaking at the same time, and it moves me to continue moving. But I shouldn't have to, and they shouldn't have to. We shouldn't have to constantly contort ourselves into twisted knots of desperation and gratitude.

EM: Thank you so much, Seyi. You've captured beautifully what a revolution that's financially resourced should look and feel like.

My last question is: If you were to imagine a future in which burnout was eradicated, what does it look like through the lens of transformative funding?

SFL: Ultimately, if burnout doesn't exist any more then I think that's because the capitalist system no longer exists. I think that's because we've been able to reimagine a world that prioritises people and not money. We'd live in a world where Level Up doesn't exist, and Project Tallawah doesn't exist.

EM: And Peaks of Colour doesn't exist.

SFL: Right. Because there's no need for them. For Level Up and Project Tallawah, our whole thing is to make sure that we're holding the people who are most marginalised, the people who are most at risk of burnout. So if burnout no longer exists, that means that those circumstances have been solved, and we, therefore, no longer have to exist either. [Pauses] And so I'm just imagining, like, green, abundant, fields where people actually get to centre joy rather than survival! A world where we're actually thinking about the impact that we have on each other, the planet, and how our actions affect the next generation and the generation after that.

EM: To come into our purpose right, instead of survival.

SFL: Mmmm. Currently it's all immediacy, right now, in the moment, and that's because it has to be, because of what we're living under. But in the future, we'll have the capacity to ask, what does it mean to *live* when we're not running for our lives? I don't know if I know the answer right now, but in a world where burnout no longer exists, I think we'll know exactly what the answer to that is.

Abundance as Resource:
In Conversation with Noni Makuyana

Noni Makuyana, alongside Guppi Bola, is the co-founder of Decolonising Economics, an organisation that strategises to move power and resources to those working to divest from a white supremacist economic model. In our conversation we discuss material resources and find ourselves in a wormhole of imagination.

Solidarity economics: a wide array of economic practices and initiatives that share common values – cooperation and sharing, social responsibility, sustainability, equity and justice. Instead of enforcing a culture of cut-throat competition, it builds cultures and communities of cooperation.[7]

Decolonising economics: A process of divesting from whiteness in order to build a solidarity economy rooted in racial justice principles. To decolonise is to contextualise, therefore, to decolonise the economy is to contextualise the capitalist economy within histories of colonialism and empire. To build a solidarity economy, we need to first understand the depth to which colonialism has influenced our modern economic system through the extraction of power and resources from marginalised communities, and the accumulation of wealth and power in whiteness, middle-classness and cis-straightness.[8]

EM: Okay, so big topics, big questions! I'm wondering if you could talk me through the ways that our current economic model perpetuates burnout?

NM: I think we burn out because these systems of oppression create a society where people are unwell. Yes, the economy is extractive, but our health, our bodies, our burnout is political, and I think it all comes down to growth. Those advocating for 'wellbeing economics' argue we can't have infinite economic growth on a finite planet. But I always think, what if we also see how the human body is finite, right? Especially as racialised people, disabled people and neurodiverse people. We're expected to always be growing, thriving, getting better and better and better and better and better at whatever cost. We're simultaneously expected to be an infinite resource, providing the invisibilised labour of undoing the wrongs of the system. But our growth is only about getting better in service of a capitalist system. So that, you know, if we were to grow more, we can work harder, spend more money. Even our growth has been commodified because we're told we can't be better unless we spend loads of money on some course. We're also not allowed to reject growth. If we want to consolidate growth, regress, unlearn, rest or feel that we're happy where we are, we're penalised. There's lots of ways in which the system puts things in place that punish us, openly or quietly, for not growing forever and ever.

There's also the monetary aspect of it, as well as social reproduction and the emotional labour of looking after your body and each other. Under this current economic system, social reproductive labour just isn't recognised, because it's always been done by Black queer, feminised and disabled people. And that is labour that the economic system would not function without. We need mothers to look after kids, carers to look after people that need care. We need people that listen, people that support us, people that do domestic labour. Without those things, the whole system would fall apart, but burnout is encouraged by that work not being valued.

People should get paid for caring roles, and jobs should also cover you to be able to have time to decompress. We know that without this you become exhausted and resentful. NGOs are a great example of this. You'll have white people, white *men*, just emailing or calling you like, 'Can you process something?' And it's like, 'I'm literally processing generations of trauma and the trauma of living in this system. I'm actually busy.' [I snort, and Noni laughs!] But it's true, I don't think we would experience burnout in the ways that we do if the invisibilised labour was valued, sustained and resourced accordingly.

EM: That feeds into my next question, which is all about resourcing the regenerative revolution. What are the things that we need – this could be material, practical, emotional, societal – so that we can firstly rest, and secondly further the fight?

NM: Universal basic income, definitely. Because then it's like, if I didn't need to work, or overwork just to meet my needs, then anything is possible, you know? I feel like being a freelancer is a taste of what that freedom could be. Since going freelance, Mondays are my self-care days. I have therapy and maybe I will treat myself to something. I like having that time and I feel like the universal basic income, and financial security, is tied to time. That's why things like the four-day working week are needed too – even though it should be a three-day working week!

EM: Yes, it should. Two days, if we're gonna shoot for the stars!

NM: Literally. Being resourced for your time and having autonomy and ownership over your time is a really big thing. Most of my family work for the NHS, where you've got twelve-hour shifts, right? Then you have a couple of hours to come home, you go to sleep, and you go back to work. You literally have no time that is purely yours. I think back to when I was working full time, compared to now when I'm a freelancer, and though I still have lots of busy periods I can really tell the difference in my conception of time, and how my brain benefits.

I also feel what we need for burnout recovery is solidarity, for realsies. Solidarity is coming together and making our dreams into reality. What the system does is it makes you individually responsible for your problems when we all have the same problem. We're all poor, we're all tired or hungry or burnt out. Burnout is how we physically realise we are all victims of the same system to varying degrees. Therefore, we all need to build solidarity around that without competition, without the Oppression Olympics. And yes, we do have different experiences but there's a need to kind of foster understanding for where we all are, without generalising experience. We *are* dependent on each other to get out of this. That means thinking how we then maintain our relationships through conflict, accountability, that type of stuff. And I think that is a really good thing, because it's nice when people are just like, 'I noticed that you're looking a bit rough, what's going on?'

EM: 'You've been very mardy recently . . .'

NM: Woah! [Laughs] It's just nice to have people care about you. Otherwise, you end up being a martyr, and that makes us burn out too. What else is there . . . [pauses] More people need to have fun in general! There should be more spaces for enjoyment and recovery. Because either you're working hard or you're trying to not be sad [chuckles]. Yeah. It's nice to have spaces to just feel that kind of connection and solidarity, spaces to gather is such an important thing. There's got to be more than just survival. Some of the organisers who come to mind who are doing really heavy work on the frontlines are also the ones who have the greatest thirst for joy, and so are having the most fun. It's a commitment to action. There's something about how we regenerate each other when we come together. And that can be quite nice.

EM: That's a lot of stuff we're missing! Even language like 'missing' makes things seem accidental. Like 'Oops, we missed your universal basic income', when these are very deliberate omissions that deny us affirming lives. We're made to believe change is so hard to implement, but it doesn't have to be. There's the top-down stuff, like UBI, but fun's definitely something we can build for ourselves from the grassroots. It's often something I take for granted, and even though Peaks of Colour's focus is on trauma, I hope our activities are still fun. I don't want people leaving sad, like: 'Oh great, I've just been reminded I'm oppressed, good one.' I want people to leave with hope for the future. Which brings me on to my last question: if you were to imagine a future in which burnout was eradicated, what does it look like through a Decolonising Economics lens?

NM: This is so unserious, but I just always think about it. You know, when you were a kid, and you would have, like, mandatory nap time? Imagine if there was just like a place where you would just pop in for a nap. Like, McDonald's, that's a bad capitalist example, Noni, but you know, it's for a nap!

EM: McDonald's but you don't wake up to Ronald McDonald — that's not relaxing.

NM: Yeah, we don't want him. Maybe we'd call it something like 'Institutions of Rest', and I guess what it would represent is one part of an economy which is built around this ethos of resting being encouraged. But also, I literally just think of futures like a great market where there's everything you need. It's fun and nourishing and you come away feeling whole and complete. Your worries about your needs don't exist because they've been met; you can go to the institute of rest and lie down because the market took care of everything for you in one spot. Yeah, that's what the future would look like, just everyone's needs being met. You won't have to prove yourself, what you need will just be available to you.

EM: I love the market idea. I'm imagining a bazaar, Marrakech-like. Everything's colourful, nice, vibrant, but then you've also got a stall where if you need a house, you go, and by the end of that conversation you've got a house! They're like, we can find that for you. Your boiler's broken? Okay, great, let's get you a plumber.

NM: That'd be amazing!

EM: A benefits stall where if you need some extra money, they're like, 'Here, have some extra money.' Imagine! All those basic needs that are really hard to access currently. Instead of having to beg DWP for money to pay your bills you just rock up to your market and Bob's your uncle!

NM: That would be the dream. And it removes the harm that all these services cause. Even the doctors init, at the market there'd be every form of healer you can imagine, and you can just go and access health!

EM: Not having to call at 8 a.m. to receive a ten-minute appointment three weeks away. Only for your GP to say they don't know what's wrong with you and they can't give you anything. It's a water infection, please give me antibiotics!

NM: [Laughing] I want all of this. Do you ever just hear something that you said, said back to yourself and you're like, wow my brain! Institutions of Rest and a Needs-Met-Market, that's what I hope for us.

Abundance as Time:
In Conversation with Farzana Khan

Farzana Khan is the co-founder and executive co-director of Healing Justice London, which builds community-led health and healing to create capacity for personal and structural transformation. Our interview takes place on a sunny July morning in Sheffield. Overlooking a pond, we watch butterflies dance among the bulrushes and talk about the ways that time is a resource often denied to many.

Temporal justice: Within a capitalist society, our time is not our own. The hours, days and weeks – including the times we are permitted rest, such as our evenings, weekends and holidays – are constructed to maximise a workforce's productivity. Temporal justice recognises that time is therefore disproportionately afforded to those with power and privilege and explores ways of reclaiming and redistributing time through, for example, seasonal, speculative or indigenous perspectives.

EM: Let's just dive straight in. Could you talk me through what temporal justice is, the issues it's resisting and why?

FK: There's lots of ways we can explore temporal justice. It's an ontological thing. Liberation is tied to our capacity to *be* because all of oppression is trying to make you other than yourself. It's really interesting because, as you know, trauma takes us out of ourselves. It either keeps us in the future, or in the past, we're never *here*. So temporal justice then becomes about being able to be in-time.

I think of Marai from Project Tallawah, just an incredible sister, beloved. She once said to our team, 'We don't have the conditions for the world that we want yet.' We're living here, where the conditions and the context are separate from where we want to be. So we have to become time travellers. And I believe that those of us who are working in trying to map out possibilities, being in visionary practice, we're time travelling. Time travelling is about our incredible capacity as Black and global majority peoples to know how to vision something better in uncertain times. Time as resource is the ability to know that the hope is legitimate, that as humans we are capable of being better and that the world can look different.

From there we can begin to ground temporal justice in specific places and contexts. For example, a piece of work that we're doing led by my incredible colleague Dr China Mills, alongside some amazing disabled activists, organisers, artists, is called 'Deaths by Welfare'. It looks at deaths and suicides caused by welfare reform. The slow violence, the chronic, sustained efforts towards the premature deaths of marginalised people. And so, we see that time is a weapon because time is lost. It's used against people, and it brutalises people.

There's another facet around the urgentocracy that we live in. The highly caffeinated [oil-reliant] petro-states, like London, where everything is linear, everything is faster, faster, faster, is out of alignment with the cyclical nature of what life is. We're seasonal. Life and death are fundamental parts of our interdependence with everything, with our ancestors, with food, with rest. I have a spiritual practice that in Islam is called Tawhid. It's a state of absolute oneness, and it's the collapse of space and time. We pray five times a day, and when you think about it, it's really anti-capitalist, because when you go to the prayer mat, you're stopping capitalist time and entering celestial timing, anchoring yourself with the sun, five times a day. Recently I was part of a space that was *stunningly* held by someone called Lisa Yancey. Phenomenal, phenomenal human being. It was about bringing global leaders together, and there was a lot to get through. But one of the things that Lisa kept saying to us as a way to stop time was 'Time is in service of us.' To hear that habitually was so important.

EM: Do you remember that kids' programme that was on CBBC, *Bernard's Watch*? For some reason that's what came to mind as you were speaking. That these practices are like our own time-stopping watch. But then we must collectively organise around these practices. Like, if you were to say to me, 'Evie, you take the time you need, I've got this', I can pause time, rest, come back to the movement renewed and ready to hold the fort for you.

FK: Exactly. Because we can't talk about rest or self-care without considering the conditions around it. One of the biggest contradictions and complexities that we're straddling is the fact that we *do* need to slow down, while also ensuring that certain actions pick up pace. I often think of my motherland, Bangladesh. We're having floods and are very much experiencing the climate crisis *now*, so we don't have the luxury of slowing down or taking our time. When I think about slowing down, it's in a way that holds an assessment of positionality and privileges. Who gets to rest? How do we build collective skilfulness and competency? Mariame Kaba says that we're tiny against the scale of might, money, resources that the Right have. So, when someone needs to slow down, they can, but the work can't stop with them. While we're building towards other worlds, worlds that we may well not see in our lifetimes, there is something beautiful about pro-portionality. I am accountable for creating many touchpoints of accountability, which to me means I'm going to pause time by being on the dancefloor every week, slow cooking once a week so I can feed myself well, taking care of my body, being in love and nurturing those relationships. We're accountable to practis-ing life outside of the capitalist binaries, and that is a real act of resistance and liberation. It's a discipline.

EM: I love the way of reframing the intention behind self-care – that my wild swimming, for example, is a radical act. One that isn't individualistic or guilt-ridden but a responsibility to pause time in service of the movement.

FK: I can just see you wild swimming and the world stopping around you in that moment! I'd also say we stop time through connection and interdependence, to interrupt a state of dis-embodied separation. It's the stopping of time towards the invitation, or orientation, of, like, absolute togetherness.

EM: The connection with the Earth, with our bodies through food, with others through dance, with the spiritual through prayer. Connection with all the relationships which have been severed through the theft of time.

FK: We went there. We time travelled.

EM: Quite literally. As you were talking, I realised I have no idea what time it is now, or how long we've been here. It's interesting – I probably wouldn't have been able to have this conversation five years ago because I was so disembodied. I imagine there's so many people at different stages of this journey and I'm wondering, could you talk me through your journey with Healing Justice so far, and what you're looking towards through that temporal lens?

FK: I guess I'll start by saying that I'm a steward of Healing Justice. That which I'm in service. I feel entrusted with a vision and the skills to steward that vision at this time. We're responding to a need, and really that need can be summarised as the recognition that when people were asking for support, there was no infrastructure that we could actually point people to, where they would not be harmed.

Fast forward to now, and we're still doing the community-oriented work that allows people to self-determine, to be present, to participate. We're recognising we need to have a structural response because of the times that we're living in, and that we have some beautiful emerging peers to be in movement with. So together we're building that capacity to be in a transformative state of *being* as opposed to a capitalist state of *doing*. This is what we're best positioned to do now – build scale. To share framework and methodology and approach and have that adapted with and worked on.

Ruth Wilson Gilmore's really anchored and given articulation to a lot of the work we're building. To paraphrase, she said: 'Abolition is not just the absence of policing, it's the presence of meaningful infrastructure.' It's the most marginalised communities that are lacking capacity, time, resources, etc, so we have three types of intervention, but also sites of reimagining: internal capacity, structural capacity and sustained capacity-building. One of the reasons infrastructure and ecosystem work is so important – and anyone who's working class or understands trauma work can relate to this – is because if your baseline material needs of safety are under chronic threat, you won't be able to regulate or repattern that trauma. This really is the next phase of what we're looking towards: building that muscle around embodied leadership, so that we know what to do under pressure, uncertainty, perpetual change. So we can consensually shape different futures through different choices.

EM: That's beautiful, thank you. My last question is one I've been asking everyone and follows this nicely: If you were to imagine a future in which burnout were eradicated, what does it look like through a temporal justice lens?

FK: I think, increasingly, it comes down to a very small phrase, which is *our ability to be in 'right relationship'*: right relationship with land, each other, all life in a way that is deeply dignifying, active, loving, tender, appropriate – not transactional, not excessive. There are communities that know how to be in right relationship, but for hundreds of years we have been removed from this knowing. We need to have a deeply interdependent global approach to this. Though there may be differences, there will be no separation between the right relationship we practise in very localised, contextualised places and the right relationship we have with a country on the other side of the world. This is how we collapse time and space, through our relationships across and within it.

EM: God, I feel so grounded. What a way to spend a Sunday morning. And the ducks appreciated it too – did you notice when you finished speaking, they all flapped their wings like they were giving you a round of applause?

FK: Look, they've come so close and are just hanging out with us. I'm so glad this happened in this way and that we could do it in person.

EM: [We stand up, and hug] Me too.

Abundance as Space:
In Conversation with Amahra Spence

Amahra Spence is the founder of MAIA, YARD, ABUELOS and countless other impressive projects guided by spatial justice and more-than-human accountabilities. Space as a resource is, therefore, the topic we delve into, and Amahra shares with us her expansive vision for Birmingham's future.

Spatial justice: drawing attention to the ways that certain demographics disproportionately experience disadvantage due to the structures of power and privilege related to geographic location. Critiquing healing and justice through a spatial perspective, spatial justice advocates for the fair and equitable distribution of space as resource and is interested in mobilising civic power on a local and regional scale.

EM: So much of your work – MAIA, YARD, ABUELOS and The Black Land and Spatial Justice Project – centres around a reclamation of space and spatial justice. Could you talk me through your journey so far?

AS: I might ask you to dance with me a little bit.

EM: I'm down for a boogie!

AS: I kind of want to go back to go forward. I always ask people about their origin stories, and I love thinking about my own. I think there were a couple of things that shaped my understanding of spatial politics. One was growing up in a neighbourhood called Handsworth in Birmingham. I would say it's impossible to not have some analysis of spatial politics and how race plays into that if you live or grew up in an area like Handsworth, because it is absolutely one of those places that has a real, significant racial history.

I'm also a hip-hop and grime nerd. These were some of the first poetic forms that were giving a vocabulary to a spatial critique. Saying that the projects, and the ends [public housing projects in the USA, or similar in the UK], are basically naff. This is what we don't like, this is what we're angry about, this is how it feeds into our relations with one another. It was speaking to spatial dynamics and the very projects that necessitated the birth of the genre. Being a child of the hip-hop/grime eras was fundamental to my own understanding of land.

I also grew up in a household where systems analysis was a default. And I think this is the case of so many – particularly Caribbean – families and communities who came over and have embedded here over two, three generations. Which brings me to the third thing: my granddad's house. As a site where I would sit at the feet of my dad and uncles having these heavy political conversations, I absorbed and developed an analysis and grew a worldview that was situated in critique, navigating and trying to stay well.

141

But my granddad's house was also this massive site of conviviality, of joy in abundance from seemingly nothingness. A house of music, laughter, comedy, dancing, performance and storytelling. I still maintain that my grandad was the first storyteller I ever met, and he's the best at it, of all time. My grandparents came over here in 1960 and landed in an area that we colloquially call the 'Black Country' because it was at the heart of the Industrial Revolution. The factories used to churn out black smoke and the soil was literally and metaphorically toxic. It was a predominantly white working-class area and so many people were struggling to find decent jobs in post-war Britain, and so the rhetoric was all about blaming the migrants for coming over and 'taking' their work. Despite that racial dichotomy that he was then placed in, somehow, my grandad still created this loving oasis. I grew up fascinated with how you could have a systems analysis that was rigorous and critical, *and* you could build loving infrastructure from that very place.

EM: I love this, and the way it shows that what can inspire a movement is already within us – our hometown, our favourite people and places, the music we love.

AS: Right! So, in 2013, when I set up MAIA, I knew that I wanted it to structurally be formed different. I knew that the physical space of where we convene is critical but for about five, six years, we were, like, popping up in other people's spaces. We were doing stuff, you know, as and where we could fit in. And it always came with massive conflicts, contradictions, tensions, things that you're weighing up, accommodating, shapeshifting.

I knew that whatever space we were going to orient toward, we had to get the conditions right. It had to allow for permanence. It has to resist the dispossession and displacement that our people have become violently accustomed to since the colonisers deemed us property and trafficked us from our home-lands – something we still know intimately in the context of, for example, gentrification. This is where we began to think of spaces as sites that build capacity for collective imagination to be materialised. What does a space look like if we become the co-designers of the neighbourhoods we live in in a non-extractive way, right? If we grow our own methodologies that speak to our commitment to one another, and the places that we're in? If we build in any way that acknowledges our more-than-human accountabilities?

EM: In the spirit of dancing, as you were talking I was reminded of your Solar System Model, and it strikes me that there are parallels between space as cosmology and space as infrastructure. Hearing you speak of it during the BAME Online panel we were both on actually inspired Peaks of Colour's developing nature-led infrastructural model, and I was wondering, well, it's not a question really, I'd just love to hear you speak about it!

AS: The Solar System idea came from thinking, 'What would it look like if the organisation could orient around the mission?' We hold the mission really tight, and hold the vision light, which means the vision is a fluid, evolving thing, but the mission is the constant. The mission is the sun. It tells you if the organ-isation is still purposeful, if it's still needed, if it's still doing what it said it would do. Around the sun – our mission – is our ecosystem, filled with our team, our ancestors, our communities. Everything affects everything else, it's all matter. It's ever chan-ging. It's planetary interdependence. Like your nature model, it's a concept that we're still breathing life into. The process of thinking what it takes to go from a solar system vision into a pragmatic organisational structure is definitely a long game. But that's part of the process of an ever-moving solar system.

EM: The power of this really can't be underestimated. I realised I wasn't allowing myself to dream of a future where Peaks of Colour could ever be the stewards of land. And now, thanks to our work with Decolonising Economics, Land in Our Names and bloody MAIA and your ABUELOS, it's all I can think about! [Chuckles]. On that note, could you tell me more about that?

AS: [Laughs] I'm sorry! So, the name of the project is ABUELOS, which means grandparents. I'm now preoccupied with thinking: How can grandad's house be the precedent for what we build? As a typology of space that other people feel an affinity to? Because anything that has been generative in any way, the government has already underfunded them, and now they no longer exist: the youth centres, the community centres, you know. Then spaces that are left don't speak to us at best – and, at worst, they actively harm us. The vision would be to take the cultural sector's hospitality budgets [because they're in the millions in the city of Birmingham alone] and build a communal infrastructure that reinvests back into the people who are culture makers in our communities. A space that feels like grandad's house.

There's a building in the community that I grew up in. This site has been derelict for about two decades, and we have our eye on it. But while we work out what it will take to acquire that building, figure out how to put it into a type of land covenant that secures that regenerative nature that we need for our communities, and raise millions of pounds or whatever [chuckles], we moved into a building adjacent so we can start laying foundations in real time. This is how YARD became a real convener. YARD is about growing, or seeding, coming together so we can start the co-visioning, building those solidarities and those connections. Can we prototype what ABUELOS would look like in its fullness on a smaller scale and generate learnings from that at the same time? I feel like my work is really about reminding us that all this abolitionist, this liberatory, this reclamation work, this land work, is spatial work. It is not a speculative exercise – it is happening in real time.

EM: This brings me to my last question! If you were to imagine a present-future in which burnout was eradicated, what does it look like through a spatial justice lens?

AS: I feel like burnout for me in a spatial justice context is coming from the perpetual racial gaslighting. There are those who constantly come to us like, 'How can we be better?', and the answer is always offered by a mass movement of people across generations who say, 'Public spaces should belong to themselves, and we should be the collective stewards of them.' We're fighting for access to space where we can attend to very deeply spiritual, cosmological, intergenerational, ancestral repair work. As communities we come together, create plans and proposals that evidence that this is possible, but are met with 'Hmm, not like that'. It's a spiritual exhaustion among only glimmers of change.

So, in terms of the in-real-time future, there's a couple of things that instantly came to mind. I don't know how well thought out they are, but we can continue dancing. I think land and property would be removed from the market. Housing wouldn't be a commodity, everyone would have a beautiful, healthy, safe, thriving space to live in. Infrastructure would be . . . I want to say public, but then I also acknowledge that not everything needs to be for everyone. More the idea of a generative land covenant over public spaces, so that they could be held for the intentions that they're imagined from, in perpetuity. [Pauses]. Yeah, I'm just like, abolish landlordism, to be honest! Oh yeah, and some type of universal income.

These are the conditions we need for that capacity-building. Only from there can dreaming . . . [pauses in thought] That's the thing with us though, the imagination work also comes from really painful places, from painful histories and urgencies. We are strong at imagining from survival. I would just love for us to have the capacities so that we could imagine from a place of abundance. From a place of genuine flourishing.

EM: That's the quote right there, bloody hell! Wow, what a mic-drop, Amahra! Thank you, thank you for all of that.

Abundance as Care:
In Conversation with Eshe Kiama Zuri

Last but certainly not least is the incomparable Eshe Kiama Zuri – activist, community organiser, doula, and founder of Co-Care (formerly known as UK Mutual Aid). Eshe and I discuss the ways that community care offers a template in which society can be resourced from the grassroots.

Mutual aid: This ensures the survival of communities through systems of shared support and solidarity. Though it can come in many forms, in Black communities and communities of colour mutual aid has looked like pardners, community education, advocacy. It was central to the works of the Black Panther Party and

Organisation of Women of African and Asian Descent (OWAAD), and the legacies are continued today by the likes of Cooperation Jackson and Sankofa 360.

Full spectrum community care: A decolonial and abolitionist praxis that embraces the wholeness and the messiness of community support. Full spectrum community care brings people together to support those most marginalised, those seen as 'undesirable' by the state. It encourages us to actively participate and work with our communities to ensure we are able to provide for ourselves the love, care, support, resources and skills we need to survive and thrive in the face of adversity and oppression. It means working from the bottom up instead of from the top down. Full spectrum community care means no one left behind.[9]

EM: Could you explain how we can understand care to be a resource?

EKZ: We're told that the only ways we can access care are through a nuclear family and failing state services. Community care as an ethos poses: What of the nurse who lives on the end of your street, and could support with healthcare needs? The tech-savvy teenager in the flat above who could help an older person with online literacy, or for that matter, any English-speaking person who could help someone for whom English is a second language navigate benefits or immigration documents. The household that has spare rooms after their kids move out that could offer shelter for the homeless person who sits outside the corner shop, or the able-bodied person who could do a grocery shop for their disabled or vulnerable neighbour. This is what we understand as care as resources, but under neoliberalism, care is something transactional, to withhold then distribute on a conditional basis. It serves no one. And means our neighbourhoods are filled with tired, burnt-out, state-dependent individuals, rather than strong, united, resilient communities.

The cruel irony is that we're told to rely on the state for care, but in reality some are afforded it and others aren't. Those who can access care often have power and privilege, while what we see is those who are uncared for will then create or join spaces due to the isolation they feel. The lack of financial and material resource afforded to movement spaces then isolates us further. As the organisers you're seen to have this more-than-human ability to just constantly give, give, give. You're viewed as a service provider and are expected to care for all the people that mainstream services discard, despite having none of the same resources as statutory institutions. It's like being martyred without permission. Community care is a collective responsibility, and it's how we resource each other without relying on the state.

EM: I find this so relatable. Holding space for a collective unlearning of this service-model mentality is something we've been trying to navigate in Peaks of Colour. That, and how to hold space for people in the community to feel equally responsible for it. Sometimes I finish a walkshop and feel so exhausted because I've spent the past however long caring for others but have felt none of that care in return. The last time we met up you were telling me about your plans to pause UK Mutual Aid due to the burnout you were experiencing, and since then it has evolved into Co-Care. Could you talk me through this journey?

EKZ: If I'm honest, the concept of 'mutual aid' became manipulated by statutory institutions during the first lockdown. 'Mutual aid' as a group became aligned with just another mainstream service, and people expected UK Mutual Aid as a group to be exactly that. It made helping those who relied on us extremely difficult, because so few people were contributing in the ways mutual aid should [taking but not giving back]. Sometimes you have to stop something before it just gets really broken. I took some time to focus on a new model, and UK Mutual Aid has since evolved into Co-Care.

Co-Care centres mutual aid as defined by Black community. My dad loves an acronym and I think I've inherited this with Co-Care. And so the 'CO' stands for Community, obviously. And then we've got the C for Collective, the A for Autonomous, the R stands for Reparations and Redistribution of wealth. And then the E is for Expansive.

Community care is an abolitionist model that allows us to create systems of care for ourselves. The intention is to begin practising community care every single day, bringing it into our neighbour-hoods, our daily acts, our politics. Understanding the philosophy that community is the most important thing. We're not talking about it from a white communist kind of perspective. We're talking about it from a radical indigenous perspective where we look after each other, centre the needs of the most marginalised and ensure that, in building something new, nobody gets left behind.

We're beginning this by focusing on building accountability through the ethos of full spectrum community care. This means we'll support people to take *and* give back. Solidarity, not charity. I don't wanna use the word 'rules' so to speak – more of a structure that supports people to have an active involvement.

EM: And structure creates safety, right? For the community, and for those holding that space, for you.

EKZ: Exactly. I'm taking my time with it, and hopefully this will help with my own burnout because, you know, it's been a whole journey for me to realise that I am also worthy of being thought about and taken care of.

This new structure should help with community burnout too, because for community care to function there needs to be people with capacity. These past few years have just shown how tired everybody is, but what tends to happen is that almost everyone engaging in mutual aid practices are rendered in need of support due to the current climate, while those who do have an abundance of capacity aren't engaging.

EM: How does it feel for you being at this stage in the process? Are you excited by the possibilities of Co-Care's next chapter?

EKZ: Honestly, no. I'm excited by the idea of care as resource and developing that further. And it's also important to acknowledge change. I think a reason that so much activism fails, and so many people get burnt out, is because we are forced – by funders, for example – to just do the exact same thing over and over again, even when we know it's not working. But I think I'm traumatised, honestly, by how stressful the past few years have been, so it's also daunting.

EM: That's understandable. But it sounds like, and feels like, the next step on a journey of actualising what resourcing care could be?

EKZ: I'm glad, because I feel like it's about having something that people will believe in and will, therefore, want to develop and grow with. With UK Mutual Aid, we wanted to help as many people as possible, but with Co-Care – whether as a continuation of this same group, or building different community spaces – it's about stripping that back and nurturing those who are also invested in community, in the politics of it, in the long term.

EM: Deepening, right? My next question is actually on the idea of the long term. If you were to imagine a future in which burnout was eradicated, what does it look like through a full spectrum community care lens?

EKZ: I'm usually a bit of a realist about things like this. I don't really like to think of utopias or what would happen in, like, the dream world, because I try to work with what we have. And I think that a very achievable step within our lifetime is for people to invest in the structure of community. This already exists in many ways. Take reparations for example – it's possible for people to begin redistributing their wealth, right now. Not just financial, but also skills. Caring resources like bringing therapy or legal advice – things that are unaffordable to so many – back into the communities.

We can also invest in things like caring community infrastructures: cooperative housing, cooperative community centres, for example, where we have spaces for shelter and to begin divesting from the external. Community care looks like having space to have these dialogues, these politics, safely without them being questioned, debated, explained. Spaces like these allow activist organisers to achieve far more together rather than feeling isolated, and I think we would see so much more grow from that. You know, this is the time for us to say, 'Okay, we're not going to fight any more. We're gonna heal and we're gonna grow and we're gonna build.'

Given the choice, I would not choose to experience the traumas that have led me to the forced scarcity of burnout. I think it's reasonable to assume that few of us would. And though the previous chapters on Exhaustion, Grief, Anger and Anxiety seek to reclaim what remains, they are also a reminder of what has been taken, of what could have been. When in community with the likes of Seyi, Noni, Farzana, Amahra and Eshe, however, I can find gratitude for the fact that my traumas have led me to such people. People whose words alone can lift me from the darkness and whose communities can warm me when the frostiness of lack begins to bite. To paraphrase the legendary rapper Tupac Shakur, the systems have got money for wars, but somehow remain unable to feed the poor. These conditions of material deprivation create a scarcity of imagination, where the impoverished margins of the status quo limit our capacity to see beyond our present conditions. These conversations remind us that this scarcity can be transformed into possibility. That with the financial and material resources, with time and space to rest, create, heal and be, and that with a community in which we are resourced through care, abundance is possible. This is not to position our suffering as redemptive, that an afterlife will reward us if we continue to suffer in dignity. It is to say that in this present-future it is possible for our suffering to become obsolete. What follows, as we will see, is joy, hope and rest. I may not be grateful to be burnt out, but I am grateful for this.

Case Study #3:
The Charity Industrial Complex

These are feminists who would say, in the
words of former political prisoner Susan Saxe,
'My feminism does not drive me into the
arms of the state, but even further from it.'
— Mariame Kaba[1]

The charity sector is the third institution I've chosen to delve into more deeply within these case studies. Those of us interested in social change are likely to find ourselves working within it, navigating it, interacting with it or resisting it at more than one point in our work. Across society, the charity sector (also known as the voluntary, third, NGO, NPO, civil or philanthropic sectors) is positioned as a benevolent force for good beyond critique. It is assumed to sit outside the state, where, we're told, external oppressions can be remedied. The reality, however, is that those of us who enter the sector, passionate and hopeful, are likely to experience and witness unimaginable harm perpetrated from inside the very same institutions purporting to be the source of help.

Across the world, the charity sector represents one of the largest global economies. The USA, for example, boasts 1.5 million charitable organisations that make up a trillion-dollar industry. Meanwhile in the UK, approximately 200,000 organisations are estimated to contribute over £12 billion a year to the British economy – equal to the agricultural sector.[2] Across Britain, the charity sector employs over 800,000 people,[3] yet in 2021 research conducted by Third Sector[4] found that 94.3 per cent of workers had experienced burnout, citing key contributing factors including the Covid-19 pandemic, poor work–life balance, funding concerns, poor organisational culture, job insecurity and the pressure to take on more work in times of external crisis. The prevalence of burnout here shows just how unfit for purpose the charity sector is.

Charity as an Industrial Complex

In *The Revolution Will Not Be Funded: Beyond the Non-Profit Industrial Complex*, INCITE! offer the 'industrial complex' (most often used to describe the socio-economic and socio-political influence of the military and prison industrial complexes) as a framework in which to understand and critique the true nature of the charity sector. A US-based organisation of radical feminists of colour, INCITE! defines the charity industrial complex (CIC) as offering a container for capitalism through 'a set of symbiotic relationships that link political and financial technologies of state and owning class control with surveillance over public political ideology, including and especially emergent progressive and leftist social movements'.[5] In other words, just as the military industrial complex profits of war and the prison industrial complex benefits from crime, the charity industrial complex sentences organisations, no matter how well-intentioned, or how in opposition to the state they wish to be, to the business of *needing* oppression, or being complicit in the state's ongoing oppression, rather than seeking to abolish it.

Food banks are a controversial example of this. Though undoubtedly meeting an immediate need, their existence has done little to rectify the rampant food insecurity across the UK, with organisations such as the Trussell Trust revealing they provided 3 million emergency food parcels across the country within the past year. This was not only their largest distribution to date but represents a 37 per cent increase from the previous year, with almost 800,000 people using a food bank for the first time.[6] Ensuring its citizens are not going hungry should be one of the fundamental requirements of the state, yet it increasingly uses access to food as a tool of policing and punishment through, for example, the welfare state. The ever-increasing prevalence of charitable solutions to such precarity absolves the government of its responsibility and validates the state's absence. In the height of the pandemic in 2020, for example, footballer Marcus Rashford fought for free school meals to be distributed to children living in poverty during the school holidays. Though the British government eventually buckled, the funds were allocated to private catering companies rather than families directly. As a result, the 'hampers' – which were supposed to cover ten days' worth of food – included only a loaf of bread, some cheese, a tin of beans, two carrots, two bananas, three apples, two potatoes, a plastic bag of pasta, three yoghurts, two Soreen loaf bars and a tomato.[7] While initiatives such as these fight the government for such meagre scraps, grassroots organisations exploring abolitionist approaches to food justice – building solidarity and autonomous communities, not charity and dependence[8] – receive very little funding and support.

While the government makes war, expands punishment and proliferates market economics, the CIC absolves the state of its responsibility by giving the illusion of care. 'A big demystifying factor of my understanding of the charity sector was learning how it came into being,' says Martha Awojobi. Martha is the founder of Uncharitable (formerly known as #BAMEOnline), a digital anti-racism resource whose focus lies predominantly on the charitable contribution to racial injustice. As Martha and I sit across from each other on Zoom, they suggest that with an understanding of the CIC's colonial legacy, this becomes easier to reckon with. 'The charity sector in the UK was essentially born from a rift between Catholicism and Protestantism during the time of Henry VIII. You had the Catholic almsgiving form of charity, which saw saving immortal souls as your way into heaven, versus the Protestant approach, which was about the impact of good deeds and, to an extent, dealing with the social ill,' Martha begins. 'Over time the individual motivation became less important than the political drive to stop a revolution, similar to what was taking place in France, happening in the UK. Charities were how the state could pretend it was actively working to appease discontent.'

INCITE! identifies that while the prison industrial complex and the military industrial complex overtly repress dissent, the charity industrial complex manages and controls dissent by incorporating it into the state apparatus. Martha agrees. They describe this system as 'philanthropic imperialism', where charities are positioned as the 'good arm' of a very violent process. 'It's like the PR wing of imperialism,' they laugh. 'And as with everything, this virtuous, moral image of the charity sector has been extremely successful in minimising and concealing England's multifaceted role in international and national violence and domination.'

Charity as State Suppression

Our present realities may seem far removed from this bygone period, yet this grounding allows us to understand the CIC's role in more recent histories in the same way – a construct that ultimately diverts would-be revolutionaries into a system where very little systemic change actually occurs. In *Race to the Bottom: Reclaiming Antiracism*, Azfar Shafi and Ilyas Nagdee evidence in detail how during the UK's anti-racism movement of the 1970s and 1980s, the CIC once again became a top-down tool that was instrumental in the state's attempts to stifle the brewing Black Power movements of the time. Largely composed of second-generation commonwealth migrants – or, rather, first-generation citizens of the British state – this movement was bold, unapologetic, mobilised and community-centred. Though not without their flaws, they challenged systems of power (employment exploitation, police brutality, anti-immigration policies, impoverished living conditions and heightened surveillance) through community organising, strikes and protests. They stood in resistance to the violent fascism of Powellism, which provided the intellectual scaffolding for what would be known as 'Britain's New Right', and later Margaret Thatcher's Conservative government, but also against the non-revolutionary politics of the left. They confronted the Labour Party about its maintenance of social hierarchies and trade unionists on the myopia of their militancy, and on an international scale they stood in solidarity with anti-imperialist and anti-apartheid struggles across Africa and the Middle East.

Shafi and Nagdee point to events of 1981 as catalysts for much of the change that followed. The state was responding with increasing carcerality and police brutality (with, for example the British Nationality Act 1981 and the notorious 'sus' laws, which permitted police to stop and search people based on a suspected intent to commit an arrestable offence). In response, racial justice groups amplified their resistance, with the Brixton Riots and the Black People's Day of Action occurring in response to the New Cross house fire, a racially motivated firebombing which killed thirteen Black children at a birthday party in south-east London. That same year, the Scarman report was commissioned. It was tasked with capturing the scope of political unrest and setting recommendations for change, but instead it dismissed the validity and severity of the Black lived experience, stating that '"Institutional Racism" does not exist in Britain.'[9] In the report, Lord Scarman posed: 'The question the inner cities raise, therefore, is are we to become a successful, multiracial nation or are we on a course for a revolutionary phase in our history?'[10] As Shafi and Nagdee summarise:

> Civil organising, as much in the 1980s as now, serves as a lid on grassroots organising. It does so by buying activists off the streets and into advocacy roles, tying them down

to the structures of funding conditions and charity laws, and reproducing a division of organising work that is shaped more by the dictates of corporate management than movement development. And, by making them accountable to funders and patrons, over the communities they seek to serve, these organisations end up forming a layer of professional activists sealed off from a popular base that prevents the formation of radical organisations. Groups whose work would have once been driven by the democratic wills of their communities become dictated by the demands of funders, and open conflict with the local and state politics grew muted as they played the fraught balancing act between seeking resources from that which they were critiquing. The political work of serving the people was subtly transformed into the task of service provision. One-time comrades came to be seen as competitors for funding pots. In this way any possible antiracist political movement is segmented both internally, and hived off from other grassroots movements externally, preventing the consolidation of a bloc that could meaningfully challenge political power, and retreating to legalistic strategies over mass organising.[11]

Rather than attempting to eradicate anti-racism directly, Scarman subtly introduced a state-led tactic to subvert the threat to white hegemony that the unwavering Black Power movement posed. The introduction of the charity industrial complex as a form of 'anti-racism from above' enacted a strategy of containment. The Black Power movement became domesticated and professionalised into a 'Black civil society' as a result. Coerced into complicity, working for the very same institutions they were once fighting, generations of Black activists have been conditioned to burn ourselves out under the illusion that the more exhausted we are, the closer we are to change, when in fact this couldn't be further from the truth.

Charity as Distraction

The CIC perpetuates an unsustainable model that positions social justice as a career done by a few overworked, underpaid and ultimately burnt-out people, rather than a mass movement of resistance built with the involvement of millions. These tactics proved to be easily translatable to the containment of other movements. As the Black Power movement was gaining widespread momentum, so were women's rights and anti-violence movements, for example. In *Abolition Revolution*, Sisters Uncut organisers Aviah Sarah Day and Shanice Octavia McBean document the movement's evolution through Britain's tumultuous political landscape, in their fight against gendered violence. Like Shafi and Nagdee, they reflect on the ways that state funding and charity modelling have been used to undercut and co-opt the once-radical anti-violence movement and organisers' visions for revolutionary change. 'We were brought up – many of us dragged up – in the post-Thatcherite landscape which had seen worker and liberation movements annihilated. As our consciousness of the world around us grew, from our childhood through to adulthood, the memory of powerful mass-organised resistance was fading,' they write.[12]

In the 1970s, the Violence Against Women and Girls sector, as we now know it, began as a rebellious network of self-sufficient squats which sat outside statutory structures, led by first-wave feminists. It's no coincidence that only four years after the Black uprising and the riots of 1981 the Metropolitan Police established the country's first domestic violence units in Brixton and Tottenham – the very same locations where the uprisings began. It's here that we first started to see survivors of gendered violence manipulated to further carceral and political agendas, with domestic violence units offering police yet more powers. 'The elite had cultivated our ignorance, engineered our movement's dependency through state co-option and severed us from our histories of radical resistance,' they continue. 'The movement infrastructure and networks of mutual aid [...] had largely been smashed, demobilised or incorporated into state structures.'[13]

While Sisters Uncut is now arguably spearheading the abolitionist gendered violence movement in the UK, Day and McBean recognise that when the collective was founded in 2014, their limited vision for women's liberation was a product of the professionalised service sector in which they existed at the time. 'Though we saw ourselves as radicals, our political horizons had been severely limited by the context in which most of us were raised,' they write.[14] It's here, I would argue, that the vast majority of the VAWG sector continues to sit today. And as a result, I would go as far as to suggest that it is no closer to eradicating gendered violence than it was in the seventies and eighties.

Much like the racial justice movement, the gendered justice movement has fallen into a pit of distraction. This is due to the same 'Equality, Diversity and Inclusion' politics, bureaucracy and funding constraints, but also by a reliance on carceral 'solutions' to gendered violences such as so-called protection orders and increased sentencing, and a relentless campaign of hate against trans communities, who are disproportionately impacted by interpersonal and institutional violence. These distractions pivot us away from each other, from our collective liberation, and towards state dependency. It harms hundreds and thousands of workers – often survivors ourselves – in the name of a greater cause, weaponising our suffering as an unavoidable consequence of the work, a self-sacrifice that we are expected to accept. We burn out, due to this contradiction in which our efforts are placed – both a gruelling undertaking which requires our urgent attention, all our energy, effort and focus, and an aspiration, where progress is slow and change is incremental.

'The entire model of philanthropy and funding feeds on and churns out urgency, with complete disregard of whether the outcome is actually helping anyone,' Martha reflects as we discuss this hypocrisy. 'We're all moving so fast there's no time to stop and think about the *real* impact. Not the arbitrary metrics and bureaucratic methods of monitoring and evaluation – which is completely meaningless on the ground and that funders use as a tool of power and control. Funders set the agenda through overseer, colonial, eugenicist, archetypal behaviour, but making organisations quantify their needs, measure their impact and fit a mould means that change can never be deeper, gradual or transformative.'

However, INCITE! recognise that while 'there is nothing we would want to save from the military and the prisons when they are destroyed, there may be much we want to save from the non-profits.'[15] The overarchingly dedicated, passionate workforce, whose misdirected urgency could be transformed into a rested, revolutionary movement, is but one example. Martha suggests that an ideological and emotional revolution is needed, one where we re-evaluate what is *actually* urgent and build from this instinctive knowing. When urgency in the charity sector is related to a colonial and capitalist idea of growth and accumulation, they say, what is actually required is degrowth. 'Imagine how our focus, our attention, our energies, our powers and allocations of resources would shift if we centred on ecological urgency, or the urgency to rest now in preparation of the fight later, for example,' they muse.

Whether it is the trauma of working within the sector that we are attempting to heal from, the mental aerobics required to protect our movements from its snare, the ways our care needs have been insufficiently met as a service user or how our collective potential for liberation continues to be curtailed by this ongoing force, for so many of us the charity industrial complex represents either a direct or indirect source of our burnout. It's here we must consider whether such a system is irrecuperable through reform, and if we are likewise calling for the abolition of non-profits. My instinct is to say, yes. Any efforts of reform constitute a distraction, and have we not been distracted enough? Instead, when we ask ourselves, *Why is the VAWG sector no closer to eradicating gendered violence? Why is the children's sector no closer to eradicating child poverty? Why are the animal rights charities no closer to eradicating animal cruelty?*, we can begin to release the chokehold that the charity sector has on us. Our liberation from burnout must not fall prey to such mechanisms. The possibilities for revolution exist beyond the limitations of such institutional forms.

On Radical Joy

We are in a time of fertile ground for learning how
we align our pleasures with our values, decolonising
our bodies and longings, and getting into a practice
of saying an orgasmic yes together, deriving our
collective power from our felt sense of pleasure.
– adrienne maree brown[1]

While working in the VAWG sector, I once asked a peer support group of Black queer survivors of gendered violence what freedom feels like for them. My query was met with silence. One person tentatively raised their hand in the circle and admitted, 'I'd like it to feel joyful, but I can't actually remember what joy feels like. Maybe I've never known.' When plagued with trauma, joy feels like an unattainable emotion. It's something you witness on the beaming faces of others, and wonder, *Why not me?* Just out of arm's reach, when we try to grab it, it slips through our fingers. For anyone whose eyes have been opened to the atrocities of the world, it doesn't sound unreasonable that joy is so hard to hold on to. After all, we live in a time of relentless crisis. Every single day contains multiple layers of political, economic and environmental insecurity, and we're reminded of the fragility of our – Black, queer, disabled, working class – mortality, constantly.

Just as a lack of time – time that is truly ours – exhausts us under racial capitalism, joy, much like rest, is seen as a luxury resource. It's accessible only to an elite few, and those who can afford to purchase joy hoard it, commodify it, then capitalise from it. The flavour of elation, soured. The rest of us are simply in survival mode, figuring out how to put a meal on the table amid skyrocketing inflation, navigating health crises in a context in which looking after ourselves feels increasingly unmanageable, putting out fires and responding to the needs of those most vulnerable while frequently neglecting our own.

Enduring abuse has conditioned me to believe that any joyful moment I may have, within a relationship or otherwise, is something to be at best sceptical of, and at worst terrified by. I have spent years witnessing with envy how a carefree happiness comes easier to my peers who have not experienced trauma. Meanwhile, the good mood my abuser may have been in would often be the precursor to weeks of silent treatment or violence. The gifts they may have showered me with would soon be used as a tool of ownership and coercion. The affection and love-bombing were never more than an attempt to mask a certain admission of guilt. Joyful moments therefore incite a sort of panic, and over time pain starts to feel more comfortable, more safe, than pleasure.

It's understandable then that feeling the sensation of joy after decades of incremental traumas can be deeply disconcerting. Joy takes us out of our heads and into our bodies, but often our bodies are not safe places to be. As bodyworker and coach Aisha Paris Smith explains, 'With the everyday pressures and threats of modern living, the naturally arising enjoyable sensations of the body are overlooked. [Yet] . . . by training our attention and focusing our mind on what feels good, we also train the body to bring more of those pleasurable sensations to the surface.'[2] And so, despite feeling uncomfortable with joy as both an emotion and an ever-increasing buzzword in social justice spaces, I find myself committing fervently to the idea of feeling more life in my body than I do death

– not least because I feel accountable to the Black Feminist thinkers, including adrienne maree brown, Aisha Paris Smith, Ruth Wilson Gilmore and Audre Lorde, who all tell me I should. This chapter invokes their intentional legacies as we embark on this earnest journey to joy.

In *Uses of the Erotic: The Erotic as Power*, Audre Lorde speaks of joy and pleasure as a gendered issue and a feminist priority. In a speech delivered in 1978, she invites us to challenge whether our perspectives on this are truly our own, or whether they've been constructed by a society that fears the power within them. Using 'erotic' as the term to describe this powerful source of knowledge, feeling, self-awareness and resistance (that can include but is also deeper than the sexual), Lorde reminds us that society teaches us to suspect this resource. Devalued, trivialised and vilified into what she describes as a 'plasticised sensation', 'for this reason, we have often turned away from the exploration and consideration of the erotic as a source of power and information, we have confused it with the opposite, the pornographic.'[3]

It is in the teachings of *Uses of the Erotic* that this chapter's exploration of joy as an embodied practice, a site of community responsibility, a source of disruptive power, and an intentional rehearsal is situated. Applying excerpts from Lorde's speech, I ask: What does joy, and therefore freedom, feel like? In what ways can we share this collective power? And what are the practices that cement this within our movement-building and in our lives?

Joy as Embodied Knowledge

> *Having experienced the fullness of this depth of*
> *feeling and recognised its power, in honour and*
> *self-respect we can require no less of ourselves.*
>
> – Audre Lorde[4]

Trauma positions joy as a myth, but Lorde counters that we can transform this incomprehensible fantasy into an evidenceable reality. The more we witness and experience joy, she says, the more we believe it to be something to which we can aspire. Its role, therefore, serves to remind us of our capacity for positive emotion, so that we can demand it for ourselves. Positioning the erotic as an embodied obligation has since furthered my interest in how we can carry it throughout every facet of our existence. It's like chasing a high I wish to remain permanent. There is no reason, Lorde asserts, why every aspect of our lives, of our work, of our relationships can't be aligned through a principle of joy. She talks of centring our practice in whatever is the answer to the question 'what feels right?' for ourselves and our communities. Our bodies know what is true and what isn't for us at any given moment, offering a certainty of self that no amount of systemic coercion can distract us from.

When there is an overwhelming amount of evidence pointing us towards fear and defeatism, I find the key to actualising this joy is rebuilding trust in it. The source of this – the thing that restores our faith in happiness – is for each of us to find, and it will come as no surprise that my capacity for this is realised through nature. One example of this is my childlike excitement of experiencing a new wild swimming spot. The joy begins to percolate with the anticipation of following a river downstream, my feet skipping down well-trodden footpaths until I reach a clearing. Here the trickling stream opens into a wide expanse. Clouds reflect upon its still waters as a warm summer sun teases us from behind them. This tranquil body of water soon drifts over a plummeting weir, the roaring sound of which muffles my giddy giggles as I set up camp. I'm desperate to be in its waters, and I can't undress fast enough. As my slow wade quickens into a plunge, I feel the waves of icy elation rise through my body. Pleasure, first in my feet, then my knees, then my abdomen, chest and shoulders. Before I know it, I am bathing in joy, and any harm, any pain beyond the safety of this enclave, feels like a distant memory. A large silhouette shadows me as a heron flies overhead and a black damselfly skims the water's edge. It is enough to send me into a fit of glee and I find myself savouring every second – a memory I know I'll need to return to on a less joyful day.

'A journey through nature is a journey back towards self, and I believe the truest sense of joy can only be found on that journey,' writes Melz Owusu, academic and founder of The Free Black University, in *Black Joy*, an anthology of unapologetically joyful accounts edited by Charlie Brinkhurst-Cuff and Timi Sotire. Discussing the ways that nature has been a lifeline for him as a Black, working-class, trans person of Ghanaian heritage, navigating institutions such as Cambridge University, Melz delves into the deeper impact that the joy of nature has on his sense of self. To experience joy in nature is not a transaction, he says, but a gift from his ancestors.

'We come from lineages of people that worshipped the land [...] this idea of oneness, and a reverence for the power of nature, can be found in precolonial traditions right across Africa and the diaspora,' Melz writes.[5] 'Nature is worthy for her beauty alone, but these spiritual and ancestral elements take us further into sacred power and joy, beyond the limits of Western science. It's a joy that our ancestors observed; perhaps they would surely be glad to know this is how we also chose to remember and connect with them.'[6]

When in a mutually reciprocal relationship with the land, nature becomes a prototype, a playground where the possibility of joy can be felt and experienced. A joy which is so alluring, we find ourselves committed to ensuring its continual thriving.

This accountability – to ourselves, each other and the more-than-human – is what adrienne maree brown terms 'pleasure activism'. Reminding us that our bodies have the capacity to hold more immense pleasure than capitalism could ever imagine for us, adrienne defines pleasure activism as 'the work we do to reclaim our whole, happy, and satisfiable selves from the impacts, delusions, and limitations of oppression and/or supremacy. Pleasure activism asserts that we all need and deserve pleasure and that our social structures must reflect this [...] Ultimately, pleasure activism is us learning to make justice and liberation the most pleasurable experiences we can have on this planet.'[7]

Establishing embodied practices in nature has been a transformative self-discipline, one that has opened me to breadths and depths of joy that ten, twenty years ago I would never have been able to have envisioned for myself. However, I have also found that once the joy of nature is experienced as an individual connection, another lesson is whispered through the leaves on the trees: *The joy of nature must be shared.* This is where Peaks of Colour was born – in the infectious desire to share the exhilaration that nature has offered me with my wider community.

Joy as Community Responsibility

> *The sharing of joy, whether physical, emotional,*
> *psychic, or intellectual forms a bridge*
> *between the sharers which can be the basis for*
> *understanding much of what is not shared between*
> *us, and it lessens the threat of difference.*
> – Audre Lorde[8]

I have often been guilty of hoping for joy to come easily, then finding myself disappointed when it doesn't. Speaking to the complexities of joy here therefore feels important. Attaining and maintaining an emotion which reaches depths of connection beyond anything superficial, fleeting or impermanent requires work, and this work isn't always comfortable. Embracing such ecstasy in spite of the unyielding horrors of the world will be contextual to time and place. Regardless, joy remains an active commitment, and we must not become idle or passive in our quest for an affirming existence.

It's my hope that any exploration of trauma that may unearth dormant emotion during Peaks of Colour's walkshops, for example, can be met with a balanced level of frivolity and fun at the surface. This requires a conscious effort to ensure that at regular junctions in the planning phase I'm asking myself, 'Where is the joy here?' And if I can't find it, I try to carve opportunities for it to grow through creative activities, conversational prompts, or a longer lunch, and with props such as Polaroid cameras, seeds or memory tins. I recognise, however, that joy shouldn't be something which is over-curated, false or forced, else it runs the risk of being inauthentic. It also shouldn't be something that one person experiences at the expense of another. As Aisha Paris Smith reminds us, 'to return to the joy of the body, we [must] come together to connect with our bodies on every level.'[9]

Yet within the service model upheld so vigilantly by the charity industrial complex, we are told that only 'service users' can be the recipients of such positive emotions. We're also told that the responsibility (or, more accurately, burden) to provide such joy must fall into the hands of a – usually overworked, underpaid and overstretched – support worker, who must pour from an empty cup to ensure the wellbeing of others. Extending joy from individual feeling to community responsibility is something we hope to espouse through Peaks of Colour. As someone who is humbly attempting to develop a skill that doesn't come naturally, however, I also acknowledge that this requires support. Luckily, when joy feels like an uphill battle, I can once again lean into a second form of trust: trust in community.

As Eshe Kiama Zuri taught us in the previous chapter, community care recognises that we all have skills to contribute to the building of a world where everyone feels held and resourced. There is no place for the lone activist shouldering the burden of being all things to all people. When joy feels unattainable for me, knowing that there is a community that can hold space for the things I may be lacking feels like a weight lifted. I trust that there is someone in the group who can bring the jokes, the banter, the dark humour that lightens potentially deep moments. I trust that someone will be the timekeeper, the pacekeeper, the person who hangs back to talk to the slowest walker, or who lets me know if the walk needs adapting to meet someone's needs. I trust that someone will be the bringer of sustenance, snacks, and additional water for those who may forget. I trust that people will listen, offer informal advice in the form of book recommendations, the number of their acupuncturist or the recipe for a herbal remedy that helps with pain. I trust that every single person in the space will bring conversation and that no one will leave the walkshop having not connected with someone else along the walk.

The ways that everyone in a community has something to offer, regardless of what official or participatory capacities may bring them to a space, is a subject that Aurélia Saint-Just and I have talked about at length. Aurélia is an embodied practitioner with Ulex, a training provider that serves social and environmental movements across Europe. In 2022 I attended one of Ulex's spaces, a BIPOC-only Regenerative Activism course set in the rolling hills of Catalunya. We spent the week in an isolated house, where we were surrounded by nature and fuelled by nourishing plant-based food. Every day we did daily exercises that encouraged learning, reflection and togetherness.

Though I had hoped to leave the retreat feeling arbitrarily 'better' than when I arrived, I had little to no expectations, an open mind and a surprising calmness. Emerging joyful was not high on my agenda, nor was it ever something explicitly promised to us. My assumption had been that what we'd learn from the space would be work-related, but I couldn't have been more wrong. Instead, the Regenerative Activism course gave me answers to questions that I wasn't even asking myself yet. The activities allowed us to engage with the most suppressed, most ignored traumas we were carrying so that happiness could be more certain in the future. What emerged from that space were lightbulb moments of deep healing and connectedness. Moments I hadn't experienced elsewhere before.

Moments like coming to the realisation that the truest way I could break the generational curse of suicidal ideation was to live. That, if nothing else, *to live is the work*. Once we choose life, the question of *how* we live, *how* our living can be affirmed, can follow. In order to actualise joyful liberation, I must first ensure I am alive. This epiphany came during an exercise that encouraged self-talk and intuitive guidance. I realised that, even on the most painful of days, by removing the choice of self-inflicted death I am ensuring that I do not impart the same pain that I experienced on those who love me. To exist is a radical responsibility.

The following spring, Aurélia and I caught up over Zoom for the first time since the course. I expressed my continued awe at the depth of introspection and interrogation that took place, and my gratitude for the three facilitators' care. Merging theory and practice alongside Aurélia, Sheila had been our political educator, and

Nontokozo had been something of a spiritual guide, having just completed a qualification in a course around ancestral wisdoms. Aurélia and the team had just finished facilitating a second training when we talked. I asked how it had gone, and whether there were any reflections that evolved with the latest retreat. Aurélia paused for a second then said, 'The two were very different, and we were surprised by this. Everything that was a learning for us was around acknowledging the level of trauma that comes with this work, and that because there is no one way it can emerge for people, we must be adaptable.'

Following the success of prior workshops, Aurélia and the team had followed a similar model, adapted only with learnings and feedback from the first with the intention of offering an enhanced experience. The contrast in how participants responded to the space was noticeable, however. They began to enter a dark space, which the facilitators spent a lot of time supporting people through: mediating conflicts, offering one-to-one support and redirecting the course to meet the needs of the participants.

'I want to really name the failings of us as facilitators in this space. We were able to turn the week around and recognise that it was time for lightness and laughter, but that doesn't mean that the first few days were not harder than they needed to be for people. As facilitators got together and realised we needed to shift the group, because we didn't want them to leave the week more exhausted, more vulnerable than when they arrived. This was never our intention,' Aurélia continues. 'A big learning for us was that joy cannot be something you take for granted. I think because the joy was so present in the first one, that's exactly what we ended up doing. I realise now that joy is contagious. It's passed onto others and then creates a culture of lightness, which I think is where the first training sat. It doesn't mean there wasn't sadness or heaviness throughout the week, but because so many participants had contributed, just through their nature, in building a container of joy, the space was able to interact with the deepness without sinking entirely.'

We talked about some of the joy-bringers in the first retreat, and I was surprised, given my discomfort, that Aurélia named me among them, citing the wild swim I'd organised after a fireside grief ceremony that was particularly emotional for us all. Similarly, one person offered a nature meditation walk one morning before breakfast, sharing their love for focusing on a leaf and marvelling at the stories it tells. Another participant, who affectionately became known as her alter ego 'Lady Bunny', would unleash all the playfulness of their inner child at regular intervals, ensuring silliness was never too far away. While another made sure that during each break there was music playing for us to dance to, allowing us to shake off any heaviness before the next session.

'Even though the emotions that arose from the second group were all valid, what we noticed was that attitudes towards the space differed between the groups,' Aurélia reflected. 'In the first course a structure began to form where everyone felt responsible for carrying the space, everybody contributed in their own way. Maybe people were feeling a little bit more free or able, or responsible to propose things and to lead things, while there seemed more resistance to this in the second group. For some reason, there was a little bit more of an expectation that we, as the facilitators, were like teachers, rather than space holders, and maybe they needed more guidance on how to contribute.'

Aurélia and I continued to talk about the role of facilitators in spaces like these, and what it is to embody joy as organisers. That we don't always have to model perfection, but in recognition of our own differing and intersecting paths, perhaps our responsibilities lie in the ways we invite people in to witness our own journey towards joy in earnest. Perhaps our primary role is to create a container in which participants feel mobilised to define joy for themselves in this space. Spaces where mutual reciprocity is nurtured, spaces that move at the speed of trust and that are directed more so by the relationships built within them than the programme we may design.

This is also how community, when cultivated with care and trust, minimises the potential for those holding the space to reach burnout. It subverts a service-model mentality that positions some as the recipients of joy and some as only the distributors. No longer are we seen only as a resource, but as someone who deserves to access the loving benefits of community too. It additionally expands the parameters of who can be considered as valuable in a space. So many of us are led to believe that activist spaces are for serious, serious people talking about serious, serious issues. But this, I believe, excludes all those whose invaluable contributions of silliness and play are overlooked. When framed in this way, suddenly we all have the potential to be activists. When we're all holding each other, there is more room for joy.

Joy as a Disrupter

> *In order to perpetrate itself, every oppression in our*
> *history must corrupt or distort those various sources*
> *of power within the culture of the oppressed* [...] *that*
> *can provide energy for change* [...] *This has meant*
> *the suppression of the erotic as a considered source*
> *of our power and information within our lives.*
> — Audre Lorde[10]

When I think of joy as resistance, as a disrupter, and a space that nurtures people to unlock that in themselves en masse, I think of

Sheffield's Migration Matters Festival. During their 2023 closing party, I found my body coming to a halt on the dancefloor. It was day nine and having attended at least one event a day, hosted a Peaks of Colour walkshop, and overindulged during Sauti Sol, last night's headline act, I was bodily exhausted. But in a good way. In an I-wouldn't-miss-this-for-the-world kind of way. And so, fuelled by fear of missing out, the promise of catered Caribbean food, and the desire to support the tireless efforts of a team whose hard work I'd intimately witnessed, I had dragged myself out of my hangover den.

The event was taking place in the converted warehouse of SADACCA, Sheffield's longest-standing African and Caribbean community centre. There I found myself joining the symbiotic wave of festival-goers. Our limbs moved as one, feet pounding the floor and hands fist bumping in the air. TootArd, an Arabic electronics duo played up-tempo, high-energy dance music on the stage. Around me, hundreds of beaming faces bounced to the beat of unbridled happiness. To my left, four members of the Migration Matters team joined arms in an embrace that turned into a spiralling, bouncing, release of ecstasy. Their eighth year, another unrivalled success. To my right, a middle-aged couple salsa danced amid a crowd of ravers, eyes locked onto each other lovingly. It was here I found my own body slowing down into a gentle sway as I soaked in my surroundings. *This is what cultivated, collective joy looks like*, I thought.

An arts and culture festival that celebrates Sheffield's historic status as the UK's first City of Sanctuary for refugees and asylum seekers, Migration Matters Festival has boasted the title of largest Refugee Week event in the UK for almost a decade. The fortnight-long festivities monopolise several of Sheffield's cultural and creative hubs to celebrate the city's eclectically diverse community, providing a platform for marginalised artists from migrant diasporas as it does so. Over the years it has featured international headliners such as Sauti Sol, Seun Kuti and Nyaruach, alongside some of the UK's leading thinkers, from Lowkey and Honey Thaljieh, to Ify Adenuga and Benjamin Zephaniah. Alongside this it fosters emergent community artists who deliver workshops and performances, pays homage to international theatre productions, celebrates traditional and eclectic music and dance, and raises awareness of the uncomfortable, pressing issues that threaten the wellbeing of our global community.

Amid a plundering of funding and resources within the arts, the existence of spaces like Migration Matters Festival has never been more vital. Within a broader socio-political climate dominated by right-wing rhetoric, we have seen how the abhorrent 'hostile environment' policies of the Conservative Party continue to further legacies of dehumanisation and persecution against those seeking refuge. While Sheffield claims to be proud of its City of Sanctuary status, it is not immune to the ways these policies translate into the everyday lived realities of local migrant communities. Only 46 per cent of residents support this status, 65 per cent of whom feel either indifferent or uncomfortable at the thought of an asylum seeker or refugee moving onto their street. Of the 2,727 hate crimes that were reported to South Yorkshire police in 2018/19, 69 per cent were racially motivated attacks, indicating that Sheffield is not always as welcoming and tolerable as this title suggests.[11]

Festivals such as Migration Matters that stand in solidarity with those most vulnerable in Sheffield have never been more significant. They platform the voices of those systematically silenced, raise awareness of the important role migration has played in shaping our cultural landscape and advocate for the continual commitment to do so across the city.[12] Though I've been a fan of the festival since its inception, it also happens to be run by my partner, who I met through working with the festival during its pilot phase. As Migration Matters evolved, so did our relationship, and over the years I have been privy to its behind-the-scenes mechanisms. This has privileged me with a much more intimate insight into the joyful ethics of production that form the festival's foundation. Void of ego or competition, decisions are made, and directions are taken based on the affirmative answer to: *Would this spark joy?*

Beyond the tired understanding that Northern creatives receive the scraps of an already meagre pot of funding and media attention, there is nonetheless an unspoken recognition that this independent arts and culture festival has the power to disrupt the status quo through joyful practice. Art in all its forms, but particularly in the forms that communicate the ways we suffer and survive, holds an exposing mirror up to the ugliness of society. Art that successfully manages to communicate the horrors of oppression through radical joy, however, has the power to incite a cultural revolution. If trauma and oppression are things done *to* us, then collective joy feels like the gift of agency and autonomy. For creatives and organisers to reject the alluring fruits of capitalism – recognition, accolades, status, ego, wealth and more – and to commit to being driven only by the pursuit of joy, can only be transformative.

Year in and year out, I witness the ways that success for Migration Matters Festival is quantified through the beaming faces of Caribbean elders playing dominoes at the back of the dance hall while teenagers fix them a plate. It's measured in the obedient *whoop-whoop*s of an audience entranced by a young Ugandan boy who, tasked with the important role of serenading an audience in his family's talent show, abandoned his duties to become the event's very own hype man. Running up and down the aisles of the venues, microphone in hand, he riffed and emceed his way to a standing ovation. It's calculated by the vibrations of satisfied 'mmm's emanating from a room of otherwise silent connoisseurs, feasting upon freshly made phở while being taken on one Vietnamese family's journey of intergenerational hunger during an audio dining experience.

Through caring, thoughtful, mindful curation, the Migration Matters team ensures that no matter your immigration status, no matter the privilege you do or don't hold, the atrocities you may have witnessed, the hostile systems you may be navigating or the burdens you may be carrying, you are able to access joy and escapism when within the walls of the festival. In the face of relentless oppressions that habitually, systemically attempt to break us into submission, this joy offers a bassy, vibrating vortex. It simultaneously protects those within and repels those outside who wish to cause us harm, sending the message that we are stronger, more powerful together.

For Migration Matters Festival, this joy doesn't end when the lights come on in the wee hours of the closing party, however. After months of curating, and weeks of relentless delivery, the team dedicates time to internal joy too. Over the years, a post-festival team day in the Peak District has become routine, with the core members, volunteers and collaborators invited to unwind with a picnic, wild swim and ball games. Along the banks of the River Derwent, which runs through the Chatsworth Estate, you'll find French jazz emanating from the Migration Matters camp, and an inflatable unicorn raft standing proudly as mascot. As an honorary addition to the team (if only in the forms of designated driver, emotional support and, occasionally, festival collaborator), what I witness on these team days is an energy that pulsates with the relief, pride and weariness of the day-after-the-night-before. For when we are able to recognise our individual and collective worth, and channel this through a principle of joy, we become our own power.

Joy as Rehearsal

Our erotic knowledge empowers us, becomes a lens
through which we scrutinise all aspects of our existence,
forcing ourselves to evaluate those aspects honestly in
terms of their relative meanings within our lives, in terms
of their erotic value. And this is a grave responsibility,
it's projected from within each one of us, not to settle,
not to settle, for what is the convenient, or shoddy, or
the conventionally expected, nor what is merely safe.
— Audre Lorde[13]

As we begin to understand that liberation is possible when we collectively orient around pleasure and longing, we build capacity for joy. Every interaction with nature, every time our sense of purpose is uplifted when in community and each moment of ecstasy on a dancefloor, are all part of a joyful practice. In our analysis of burnout, we can apply the teachings of Ruth Wilson Gilmore, and subsequently Healing Justice London, who offer the concepts of 'rehearsals' and 'rehearsing freedoms'. This is a way of understanding these experimental, explorative ways of collectively envisioning and practising futures free from oppression. 'Rehearse the future, rehearse the social order coming into being, as against [...] the complaints or the demands for that other path, the one that [we] don't want to take anymore,' Gilmore says.[14]

When I think of rehearsals taking place in the outdoors, I think of Ingrid Pollard's 'Pastoral Interlude'. Pollard is a photographer of Guyanese heritage whose works on race and belonging in the British countryside interrupt preconceived notions of nature and its perceived Britishness. 'Pastoral Interlude' is a series of photographs taken in 1987 portraying Black people in the Lake District. Throughout all the images there's an overall sense of unease and discomfort between the subjects – who are meditative and self-protective – and the landscapes they interact with. In the first image, for example, Pollard's subject perches on a drystone wall, a camera resting on their knee. Behind them, barbed wire lines the horizon against an undulating landscape as they face away from Pollard's gaze in contemplation. It is as if they have been captured in a moment of realisation that in the countryside all we are permitted to be is a surveyor behind human-made barriers.

Each scene in the 'Pastoral Interlude' series is accompanied by a lyrical caption, which serves as a footnote that disrupts the long-standing narrative that the countryside is unquestionably idyllic and aspirational: '. . . it's as if the Black experience is only lived within an urban environment. I thought I liked the Lake District; where I wandered lonely as a Black face in a sea of white. A visit to the countryside is always accompanied by a feeling of unease; dread . . .'[15] reads the first. Through these captions, Pollard highlights the contradiction of emotion felt when in nature: the serenity of collecting shells at the coast is met with the haunting reminder of how the sea holds the souls of enslaved people, and even when granted access, a Black face on the 'green and pleasant lands' owned by white landowners still feels like trespassing.

There is only one photo in the series that conveys an overt element of playfulness, where a person walks along a wall, arms extended as they steady themselves. That the wall frames a graveyard, however, offers a metaphor for our ability to play and to access joy, and of the way we might balance the grief of the past and the childlike desire for awe and wonder. A superficial examination could therefore infer that Pollard's images do not portray joyful scenes at all. This, she says, has been a common misinterpretation. In a *Guardian* interview, Pollard recounts how the pictures were in fact taken while on holiday with friends, and how they capture happy moments. 'People immediately say [about 'Pastoral Interlude']: "It's about alienation. It's about white landscape, Black people. It's eerie" [...] People want me to say that I'm alienated,' she reflects.[16] What the pieces actually depict, Pollard explains, is a lifelong engagement with the British land-scape in all its complexity. The text and images are in opposition to each other and speak to the negotiations that are required of people of colour as we practise and prototype what it is to be joyful. Many truths can be held at once; we are both the carriers of generational wounds and the recipients of, and curators of, happiness in nature.

Our communities have, after all, been creating joyful art from our pain for centuries, but we are told there is a time and place for our culture, and the outdoors isn't one of them. There is a cookie-cutter shape of an 'outdoorsy person' (someone kitted out in expensive, branded gear, marching intently to beat personal bests as they *conquer* the land) that we're made to feel we should emu-late. POC-run outdoors groups like ours are expected to assimilate into this image. Rather than 'diversifying the outdoors', however, Peaks of Colour seeks to decolonise it, and through Pollard's work we can find inspiration for the many variations that a 'Pastoral Interlude' can present as. Not only by our mere presence in the outdoors, but also in the ways we subvert the normative narrative of what it means to interact and grow intimacies with nature.

When I think of the subtle, everyday pastoral interludes I have been fortunate enough to witness through Peaks of Colour, I think of Noni's bright orange faux fur coat, impractical and certainly not waterproof, that she bounced around in during a Decolonising Economics woodland walk. I think of Udit, a former Sheffield resident, who rode through the suburbs and green spaces that connect our Green City to the Peak District playing Bhangra and Bollywood music on a bicycle modified to incorporate a speaker. And I think of two Southeast Asian men, whose names I no longer recall, who my friend and I happened upon one afternoon. They had taken a six-piece cooking set down to the local river, and were offering homemade kebabs, cha-pattis and friendly conversation to anyone who passed by their fireside campsite.

These are all ways we rehearse the joyful every day by building relationships with nature on our terms. Likewise, we interpret Pollard's series as what this intentional practice of joy-making could look like through a photographic medium. Originally captured in black and white, the five images were hand-tinted using a gelatine-silver print. The rejection of monochrome here can be interpreted as a reflection on what it means to purposefully bring colour to our lives. These pieces speak to the everlasting journey of being seen and seeing ourselves resting joyfully in the outdoors. Be it Pollard's photographic moments of the past or Peaks of Colour's walkshops taking place in the present day, over generations communities of colour continue in this legacy of joyful rehearsal. Redefining and reimagining what joy – within our respective time and place – looks and feels like. This, as Lorde prophesies, allows us to know in our bodies that we are capable of feeling positive emotions, that we have the capacity for joy, and that we can claim it in all aspects of our lives.

Centring joyful practice in this way makes us unruly. It makes us ungovernable. An act of healing and resistance combined. Both Gilmore and Lorde talk of the importance of observing which of our endeavours succeed and fail in bringing us to our fullness, to our joy. With this awareness, we can identify too what it is we're leaving behind – whether that's the conditions which facilitate our burnout or a white supremacist construct of nature connection. And, through joyful rehearsal, we can orient ourselves towards the future we truly desire, even if we don't quite know what that looks like yet.

On Radical Hope

Say these words when you lie down and when you rise
up, when you go out and when you return. In times of
mourning embroider them on your garments, tattoo them
on your shoulders, teach them to your children, your
neighbours, your enemies, recite them in your sleep, here
in the cruel shadow of empire: Another world is possible.
— Aurora Levins Morales[1]

In January 2023, a series of Zoom calls took place between myself and Chelsea A. Jackson, in which we spoke about hope in its many forms. In a relay of deep conversations, and even deeper belly laughs, she first questioned me as a guest on an episode of the *Post-Woke Podcast*,[2] which she founded and hosts, and I then put Chelsea in the hot seat as an interviewee for this book. A jack of all trades in the realm of transformative justice, Chelsea is a scholar, activist, speaker, strategist, facilitator, consultant and member of Cradle — a collective of activists and artists seeking abolitionist responses to systemic violence. This is how we first met, at a Cradle-led workshop on bystander intervention, which had taken place in Sheffield the previous summer.

Chelsea begins each episode of the *Post-Woke Podcast* by explaining that 'being post-woke is just like being someone who's just woken up from a long nap: aware, annoyed and activated. Aware of social issues like racism and the climate crisis, annoyed at the systems that keep them in place and activated to do something about it, creating a different future.' She asked me what my awakening moment was, and I explained how, in the VAWG sector, the goals of abolitionists – that is the eradication of conditions which see carcerality and policing as the solutions to social problems – always felt like an unrealistic ideal. It's nonsensical that the sector positioned as responsible for the fate of survivors should discourage dreaming of anything as ambitious as the eradication of gendered violence. The reality, however, is that when trapped within the trenches of frontline support, your aspirations are reduced to the primal: wishing for the survivors you support to still be alive when you get to work the next day – or that, as the support worker, you make it through the day without crying. This hopelessness meant that I had gradually become disenfranchised from and disenchanted by the work. Upon leaving, however, I experienced an almost instantaneous relief that felt not too dissimilar to the anticipation of freedom I felt when leaving my abuser once and for all. This was my epiphany.

When Chelsea and I hop back on Zoom a few weeks later, with me wearing the interviewer hat this time, we continued our musings on hope and hopelessness. 'Last time we spoke,' Chelsea recounts, 'you said burnout sits on the intersection of working tirelessly for something you're passionate about, and feeling that no matter how hard you fight, the injustice still remains. Any progress in the face of said injustice feels minimal and disproportionate to the energy it required. That really stuck with me. It's feeling like you're not having an impact. You're not seeing the needle move.' She gives an example of police brutality, both in her home country, the USA, and here in the UK, where she currently resides.

'Every time someone gets killed by police, there's protests, we go out on the streets, we say this is unacceptable. We say police bias exists, and therefore we need police reform, we need Black police officers, we say they need body camera training. Then they kill another Black person. And we go again.' Considering the disillusionment that comes from reformist politics, Chelsea relays a conversation with her dad that was the catalyst for her own awakening. She recalls how palpable her loss of hope was, that she told him she was tired of fighting, of being angry and hypervigilant, and of feeling like they were losing every battle. 'He told me: "You keep talking about all the things you're fighting *against*. But what are you fighting *for*? Because if you don't know what you're fighting for, then it's always going to feel like you're losing."' She smiles. 'My dad made me realise that if you don't have abolition, your work is only in destruction, and there's no hope there. That's what's draining. No one is manifesting the demolition. The tearing down is just what happens before we build those hopeful futures.'

It is in the scaffolding of these hopeful futures where this chapter sits. Among the wreckage of a crumbling society in which hopelessness is ever present, we must begin to construct a tangible vision for change. Under white supremacy, our visions have been constrained by its decaying parameters. An article I wrote for Refinery29's *Unbothered*, while still working in the VAWG sector, is a perfect example of that. In it, I advocated for 'burnout leave' to be a contractual obligation that employers should uphold. And while it's not an altogether terrible idea, I now see how my desires for rest were confined to the limiting margins of racial capitalism.

With my abolitionist awakening officially established, I found myself hoping for more for myself, and for others, than to simply be given more time off from our harmful workplaces. I wanted the absence of burnout entirely and understood that for this to be actualised we must build a future in which we are no longer fighting. We are no longer fighting because there is nothing to fight. In this future, oppression and exploitation don't exist and our only task is maintaining and amplifying the justice and love that has prevailed against harm and hate. I can now confidently say I know this is possible. I know this because I'm surrounded with others devising reality from their dreams every day. I know this because I am one of them.

Hope as Experiments in Imagination

It's only rational, however, that so many of us should feel so routinely hopeless. I often find myself numbed with despair as seemingly every headline reports the gradual erosion of our freedoms. I believe that our communities possess a generational knowing, that no matter how bad things may seem to be now, or conversely what improvements that have been made so far, our circumstances can always get worse. It's the inescapable burden of comprehending the magnitude of what our ancestors survived — or didn't survive. No matter how feverishly systems of whiteness attempt to erase our history, we know this to be true.

Yet to have radical hope means to believe that our destinies are *not* pre-written, despite this ever-present precarity. Complementary to Black Feminism, Afrofuturism — an artistic, theoretical and organisational praxis that transforms speculative narratives into hopeful depictions of a liberated future — provides expansive visions which ensure that *everyone* is emancipated from the chokehold that is a capitalist white supremacy.

Science fiction writer Octavia E. Butler, for example, proffers some rules for predicting the future. One of these is, aptly, to learn from the past. She warns us to not be rendered inactive by history's predictions and that 'wishful thinking is no more help in predicting the future than fear, superstition, or depression.'[3] Similarly, Lola Olufemi, writer, researcher and member of the Bare Minimum Collective, positions hope as a 'commitment to see through, around, and beyond unending misery [...] to remain steadfast in the belief that this cannot be all there is.'[4]

Tina Campt, theorist of visual culture and contemporary art, adds to this pedagogy, stating: 'The grammar of Black Feminist futurity is a performance of a future that hasn't yet happened but must [...] it is the power to imagine beyond current fact and to envision that which is not, but must be. It's a politics of prefiguration that involves living the future now [...] as a striving for the future you want to see, right now, in the present.'[5] Meanwhile, educator, abolitionist and grassroots organiser Mariame Kaba simply reminds us that 'hope is a discipline'.

Hope is a verb. A doing word. We are hopeful because we are being, because we are acting, because we are participating. Our confidence and optimism are reinforced, upheld and re-established through constant practice. And it is in this action that the joyful speculative comes into being. In the inevitable moments where our hope wavers, we are then able to turn to the community gardens, the archivist initiatives, the political education spaces, the prison abolition campaigns, the sustainable energy projects, the Mad Prides, the transformative funding alliances, the mutual aid cooperatives and the grief circles, and be reminded that it's not all pain and suffering.

Together, hope and imagination are infectious; they expand and grow and multiply. I've found that once you imagine something, you create it, and you realise this thing that white supremacy told you was unfathomable is in fact possible. Your existence is living proof of that possibility. Then, you can't help but dream further. You permit your hope to extend itself in directions whose visibilities were once blurred to you, chasing the ecstasy of the unknown and, lo and behold, you find more *what-if*s, more alternatives, more experiments, more *shall-we*s.

This is why one of Peaks of Colour's core principles is 'Experimentation' – a hopeful politic in practice. In fact, we consider every direction we take to be an experiment. When you're working to build something that doesn't currently exist, where there is no road map to follow or template to copy, how can it not be? Some of Peaks of Colour's experiments are everyday, like exploring whether we feel more mobilised and focused in team meetings held in cafés, homes, outdoor spaces or in transit on a walk. Some experiments are more personal. I'm constantly testing the boundaries that my own healing places on my leadership, for instance. Others are communal experiments, such as our aforementioned seasonal practice of going into hibernation during the winter months. We liked that one, and it stuck.

Structural experiments may look like seeing if we can exist without becoming a constituted organisation – we can. Others may require more negotiation on our part. Our original assertion was that we wouldn't take any money from white funders, for example. We've since negotiated our position on this so that if we do accept money from white-led funders, it's on *our* terms and they meet *our* criteria. Similarly, we originally resisted getting an organisational bank account, but when we realised that we could access more money than we'd ever imagined (and more money than I was comfortable holding in a personal savings account) we relinquished. As an unconstituted organisation, however, there was only one bank we could find to host us. Yet if we had been unsuccessful in securing an account with them, it would have been fine. We'd have experimented with other forms of economies.

In our work, our activisms, our homes and our communities, we are all navigating certainties that have been dictated to us but don't always sit comfortably. In every inevitability, however, there are options, opportunities for investigation. Naturally, these experiments often fail or, rather, become lessons learned. At Peaks of Colour, we have found that some come with risks, others with unpredictable rewards. Many of these experiments are ongoing and will remain a constant process of adaption. Some may be paused momentarily as an idea incubates while we figure out our next steps. And, so, we embark on slow but intentional wayfindings, with an openness to change and the possibility that the journey may itself allow the outcome to evolve. Either way, this excursion will be therapeutic, it will be thrilling, it will be fun.

Under racial capitalism we are told that our aspirations for this work must fit neatly into the corporate criteria of 'monitoring and evaluation' that funders so often subject us to. Lola Olufemi, however, describes the 'otherwise' as something empirically unquantifiable, but which can be felt, heard, touched and tasted, 'a firm embrace of the unknowable; the unknowable as in, a well of infinity I want us to fall down together.'[6] The sheer creativity of an experimental practice such as this not only negates so much of the potential for burnout that exists in the rigidity and conformity of the status quo, but it also allows us to rid ourselves of the shackles of perfectionism. If we can resist outcome-oriented organising, and therefore embrace the discomfort of imperfection, then the messiness and the mistakes can become a part of the process and the possibility. Our commitment to imaginative experimentation allows us to let go of the grinding weight of responsibility that so often comes with feeling that hope is dependent upon us getting it 'right' first time. Rather, it is our relational solidarities – that is, the ways our liberations are interconnected and interdependent – which offer us the answers we seek, 'reveal[ing] the plurality of the future-present, help us to see through the impasse, help temporarily eschew what is stagnant, help build and then prepare to shatter the many windows of the here and now'.[7]

When I started Peaks of Colour, it was from a place of burn-out. I refused to even contemplate the potential for it to be bigger, deeper than the original offer of one walk a month. My imagination was merely stagnant water. Now, it overflows, a voluminous source of inspiration and excitement, flowing in directions so adventurously that I simply cannot contain it. There is much to be hopeful for, to build towards, and it is largely those relational solidarities that ignite it. Our work with and proximity to Decolonising Economics, Land in Our Names and MAIA, for example, has urged us to dream of one day being stewards of our own plot of land in the Peak District. In this hopeful future, we foresee a stewardship that is shared by other abolitionist and artist communities of colour. A space that not only allows us time and space to imagine and build, but also, imperatively, to rest and simply be in community with each other. This experiment is still in its dream-state, and we don't yet know how we will actualise it (if any rich, white landowners in the Peaks are reading this and are looking to pay reparations, come through), but all I do know is that in the moments where my mind quietens to a hum, I find myself scribbling poorly drawn sketches of floor plans of this imaginary future home. The seeds have been sown.

Hope as a Black Utopia

Our work with and proximity to RESOLVE Collective offers another example of the way relational solidarities have permitted hope to infect our organising. RESOLVE Collective is an interdisciplinary collective that incorporates design as a tool for political and socio-economic change. Combining architecture, engineering, technology and art, their work aims to produce new knowledge and ideas, centring those who have been marginalised. During the summer of 2023, we joined RESOLVE for their Nurturing

Ecologies residency. Spanning eighty hours over the course of seven days, with forty participants, fifteen workshops, thirteen community meals and two nights out, the residency took place across some of Sheffield's most prominent activist spaces: galleries, community centres, DIY event spaces, cinemas. Each workshop was led by a different participant of the residency, meaning we were able to sample an array of practices that were as expansive as they were deepening.

It's difficult to capture the experience in words. Intentional. Hopeful. Energising. One evening, after the final workshop of the week had come to a close, founder of Healing Justice London Farzana Khan described the week as being 'breathed into', and that feels pretty accurate. Life-affirming. Life-giving. Life-expanding. 'You called and we answered, we dropped tools and came running,' she continued. She's right. No matter how busy our personal and professional circumstances were, every single person who received an invitation did what they could to ensure they were physically and emotionally present in the space. We took time off work, we came straight from airports, we found childcare, we rearranged plans, we rallied round on the days when we didn't feel our best to follow an intuitive knowing that the only place we needed to be was at the Nurturing Ecologies residency.

Though every single second spent in and among the residency felt like a homecoming, there were two aspects in particular that shone a bright light on the true impact of operating within a community rooted in a hopeful politics. The first was undoubtedly the fact that it was hosted in Sheffield. Though our city often feels overlooked and underestimated, at the start of the residency a Radical Black History tour, led by the late historian Mark Hutchinson, reminded us of its enduring legacy of grassroots activism. Mark's tour of a city that Frederick Douglass, Malcolm X, Olive Morris,

Paul Robeson and Ida B Wells frequented, left us revitalised as we began the week with a feverish sense of space and place. For those new to Sheffield, it cemented our relevance within the racial justice movement. For those of us fortunate enough to call Sheffield home, we were able to roll out of bed and witness our city as the source for radical potential for change that it is. This completely renewed my sense of belonging. So often those of us in the North are told that true safety, true solidarity, true revolution, true respite is only possible over *there*. London, for big community events. Wales or the Lake District for retreats. I had never considered the impact this may have on our own relationship with home.

The second deeply transformative feature of the residency was the peer-led element. The impact of this wasn't immediately obvious to me, rather it was a reflection that came during a long car journey as I was trying to communicate the sheer immensity of the week to my partner. It was here I realised that, rather than being a coincidence or a nice feature of the programme, the ways we all contributed to the programme were foundational to its soulful success.

To be given the opportunity to share not only people's practices, but to experience their passions, what gets them up in the morning, what alights the hopeful fires in their souls, what makes life worth living for them, what makes this work worth it, is to be invited into a depth of connection that few of us can replicate day to day. So often our artistic and activist practices are forced to contort into structures of depersonalisation. A Zoom meeting here, an email thread there. A short-term collaboration, a panel discussion, a social media connection. No matter how much we've interacted with each other's work previously, admired it from afar, engaged with it in piecemeal settings, it is impossible to achieve a sense of intimacy and trust in these ways. The peer-led structure of the residency fostered this beautifully, however. Within but a few days we became deeply comfortable with one another, tactile, homely, able to speak our needs and know they will be met, able to show up as whichever version of yourself and know the group would not only hold you but transform your mood for the day, able to feel like only the confinements of that space mattered in the moments we were in it. We fell in love with each other quickly. That's how it felt. Like falling in love.

This connection also went beyond an opportunity to simply get to know each other better. Rather than a traditional teacher–student dynamic, at no point in the week did we feel like we were merely witnessing individuals relaying their work. Instead, with each practice shared we got closer and closer as a collective, slowly enmeshing into a symbiotic whole, in which all respective practices were inspired by, informed by and evolved through the lens of each other's passions. Hope wasn't something we had to consciously curate here. Through this love alone, anything felt possible. One example of this was the workshop delivered by Nathaniel Télémaque – a self-described 'friendly neighbourhood' visual artist, researcher and writer, whose work centres around urban settings and the everyday.

Nathaniel had asked us all to submit a couple of photos that we had taken throughout the week. When we arrived at the workshop, we were presented with our photos, printed out and laid across a series of tables. In the centre of each table were empty scrap-books and photobooks which Nathaniel was offering as inspiration for us all. He introduced us to his sequencing practice, a form of storytelling that through the ordering and reordering of images allows him to create new narratives in his work. This was our task today, to take our experiences and collage them into new meanings. Nathaniel's only instruction was to have fun with it, and together we set to work experimenting based on theme, timeline and colour scheme.

With the support of Nathaniel's practice, and his captivated interest in my own writing process, I was able to acquire a lens through which to better understand the narrative and story I was trying to tell when writing this book. I was able to experiment with forms of sequencing, sitting with what felt comfortable and challenging myself to sit with the formats that didn't, until I ultimately came to understand myself as someone who views the world, and my words, through a thematic sequencing lens. Hence each chapter here being based on an emotional aspect of burnout. It gave me purpose, structure and confidence in the contours of my writing. A map to follow in the overwhelming moments. Knowing this allowed me to apply an intentionality to the storytelling in the very book you have in your hands right now.

In Nathaniel's workshop I was also gifted the opportunity of seeing Peaks of Colour through the eyes of others in the space. The day before, I had led the group on a walk through the Peaks, and photos taken during the walk were used in Nathaniel's workshop. I watched as people collaged images based on the alignment of horizons, based on how the images made them feel, based on the subversion of image to message. I had to leave the session early to go to therapy, and just as I was saying my *see-you-later*s, someone shouted, 'Wait, Evie – come and look at what Rosa's made!'

Arranged on the table were a selection of six Polaroid photos, all taken from the walk in the Peaks. In black marker pen, inter-disciplinary artist Rosa-Johan Uddoh had annotated under each image: *WE HAVE NOTHING TO GAIN BUT OUR FREEDOM!* 'You know the June Jordan quote, "We have nothing to lose but our chains?"' Rosa asked me. I nodded, speechless. 'That's the first thing that came to mind as I was laying the pictures out. But it just didn't resonate with Peaks of Colour, and so I thought, maybe Peaks of Colour is the next chapter in the story, the part of the story where we're all free, and well . . . here you go!' She gestured across the table, and, after receiving a hug from me, began taping the images into the scrapbook, assured and content with the final outcome.

Through a sequencing lens, both Rosa and Nathaniel offered a hopeful invocation for Peaks of Colour's work. A reminder that freedom is what we are longing for, working towards, and that this experimental, creative, imaginative process can itself be freeing. These are but a few examples of how RESOLVE's Nurturing Ecologies residency helped me articulate an absence of something I'd felt but couldn't previously name. It was the ability to see, feel, experience and live revolutionary everydays. Something tangible. That electric, agitated excitement where your needs, visions and practices align and are actualised. It left me with many questions that support us to toward actionable hope:

> *What freedoms lie in wait if we divert from well-trodden paths and embark on a different route?*

> *How can Peaks of Colour's everyday practice feel revolutionary?*

> *What if our Green City was a Black Utopia?*

Hope as Fugitive Futures

Writer and professor of African American studies Saidiya Hartman says how 'so much of the work of oppression is policing the imagination.'[8] It's for this reason I believe it's no accident that communities of colour in the West are as disconnected from the land as we are. Recently scientists have confirmed that spending time in nature increases our propensity for both hope and creativity, but why would our oppressors want us to have the time and space to imagine, let alone create, our own freedoms? Wouldn't they rather us be burnt out, exhausted, disillusioned and under-resourced, pre-occupied with our ongoing survival rather than pending liberation? Meanwhile, we continue to live in the legacies of a white imagination. An imagination that has the boundless ability to design a society in a racial capitalist vision. The white imagination contains and curtails the abundant parameters of our joy, hope and rest, restricting our abilities to imagine beyond an oppressive status quo. It creates borders, prisons and institutions that maintain power hierarchies and destructive hegemonies. It decides who gets to be free, and who must remain unfree. So often, our hopes for ourselves, for each other and the more-than-human are mere requests expended in mid-air by faceless agents of whiteness – funders, managers, governments. These agents make promises that when rescinded have the ability to short-circuit revolutionary experiments, dampen radical imaginations and leave material consequences for the present-futures to which we aspire.

My own exploration of imaginative experimentation has led me to the underground worlds of fungi. Fungi are a diverse array of organisms that live mostly out of sight, and what we typically know to be fungi – the bulbous, bouncy mushrooms that we find nestled deep within our forests, are simply only the above ground part of the organism. Though we know that fungi are integral to plant growth, helping them to draw water and nutrients from the soil, their full capacity and power is unknown. As a result, research is being conducted into fungi at a colossal rate, looking to uncover how they may be able to support a range of issues, from organ transplants to biofuels to construction.

One such expert contributing to the research is Maymana Arefin, the founder of *fungi.futures*, a fungi-guided space that through plant and fungi walks invites others to experience their extraordinary world. In 2020, Maymana's award-winning MSc research – conducted during the Covid-19 pandemic – established how the mycelial networks of fungi, in particular mycorrhizal fungi (the ones that connect with tree roots and plant roots), can be used as a metaphor for mutual aid and community care. Maymana described how fungi transports and redistributes nutrients between organisms, ensuring an equilibrium across ecosystems, where every organism has what it needs to survive. This, she noted, drew strong parallels with the agile and web-like ways that mutual aid networks share lifesaving support, resources, safety and information. Reciprocal actions building systems of hope through times of uncertainty.

Maymana's work is a testimony that offers a fascinating insight into the transformative connections that can be made between the human and non-human world. It evokes a sense of awe and wonder and of possibility, something Maymana underlined in their research: 'I began this work from a place of grief and finish it with a renewed sense of hope.'[9] It was this feeling that we wanted to emulate in our Reimagining Fugitive Futures walkshop, which was inspired both by Maymana's work and Black Feminist Akwugo Emejulu's concept of fugitive feminism.

Fugitive feminism has a wide-ranging definition that seeks to reclaim what it means to be 'human'. Emejulu details how, under racial capitalism, 'the human' excludes anyone who doesn't meet the hegemonic binaries of race and gender – a status or categorisation which marginalised ethnicities and genders will never be able to attain, no matter our attempts at inclusion. 'To believe I am non-human does not mean I believe in my own inferiority. Rather, it means I believe that the human is a construction of whiteness and any discussion about Black inferiority is a product of the futile struggle to be recognised as human,'[10] writes Emejulu. This, she cautions, is a distraction. And while there is grief involved in coming to terms with our own un-humanness, embracing our fugivity exposes a well of hope and possibility.

Acknowledging fugivity to be a wild proposition, 'a paradoxical experiment to see whether it is possible to embrace the fugitive's porous, shifting and unstable identity for a Black Feminist liberation,'[11] Emejulu asks: 'What would it look like to generate relations of care and solidarity with those Others outside the category of human?'[12] and how might we instead begin to understand ourselves as being 'in community and in relation with other lives on this planet — both inside and outside of oneself — as part of an ecological system'?[13] And so it was that we began our Reimagining Fugitive Futures walkshop on a Saturday in September, full of the radical possibilities entailed in this alternative view of the human and non-human.

The walkshop invited participants to explore worldbuilding through a foraging expedition led by Maymana, and a nature-allied art workshop led by interdisciplinary artist Bryony Benge-Abbott. During an unseasonably sunny morning, Maymana guided us through Ecclesall Woods, a forested enclosure situated in the Sheffield suburbs. Time stood still as they introduced us to birch polypore and its antimicrobial properties, puffballs and their pixie dust-like spores, wood hedgehog with their spiky undercarriage and earthy scent, 'dead man's fingers' and the ways their latex-like exteriors wrap around the nature they encounter in a supportive hug, and the communicative power of slime moulds which inspired us to consider the ways we resource each other in community.

It was in between meetings plotting and planning this walkshop that I sat down with Maymana and spoke to them about their practice. I asked them what we could learn from nature about creating thriving ecosystems amid so much ecological and societal burnout. 'I think the key to that question is what we can *learn*, not what we can *take*,' they responded. 'A worrying trend I've noticed in conversations around fungi is that people are like, "Fungi are the future, fungi have all the answers." There's a toxicity in that. I do deeply believe that we have a lot to learn from fungi, and from nature more broadly, about how we heal. But I think there's a real desperation to find something that will heal us, that counteracts the role capitalism's played in creating the problems in the first place. I guess a tangible example could be the ways that fungi are used for soil remediation, even soaking up oil spills. They're recruited almost to solve these huge disastrous events that are happening because of big oil corporations and gas corporations, and all that is doing is recreating the same cycles of extractivism to *serve* capitalism. When actually there is so much potential to learn from fungi tools to *resist* capitalism.'

'I'm constantly amazed and awe-inspired at how the mycelium, especially mycorrhizal fungi, have the resilience to regenerate, and find a way within the soil to connect,' Maymana adds. 'Even amid the plundering of the forests and the destruction of soil, they still can find connections and create this amazing web to redistribute resources. That's obviously so hopeful to me.' And they're right. As Maymana's research evidences, we often see how movements move like mycelium, especially in the most oppressive of times. The Underground Railroad – a network of secret routes and safe houses established by abolitionists which helped enslaved people escape during the nineteenth century – also springs to mind as one such example. Against the backdrop of a political landscape of increasing fascism, where so many of us are struggling to meet our basic needs (including our basic need for connection and rest), the template of mutual aid and community care that mycelium provide reminds us that we can look to our natural world for the hope that we need to continue. And when we see ourselves as part of a wider ecology, we are able to recognise our non-human account-abilities – not in service of a capitalist hegemony, but in service of building a future where all life is cared for. 'Fungi forces us to ask, how do we build structures and mindsets that will shift our behaviour in ways that feel more conducive to solidarity and show-ing up, without necessarily expecting anything back and without allowing our egos to get in the way?' Maymana says.

I ask Maymana a personalised variation of one of the questions that I've posed to every interviewee: If you could imagine a future where burnout doesn't exist, what would it look like through the lens of mycelium as mutual aid? They start beaming, swaying restlessly as I waffle on with unnecessary context. 'The reason I'm smiling is because I was just thinking about how it would be a place where everyone's needs are met, and how huge that would be in terms of, like, how far away from our current reality it is,' they begin. 'Especially through a mycelium lens, it would be replicat-ing the ways of the forest: the kind of call-out when an individual tree is struggling for example, and how the surrounding ecosystem immediately starts diverting resources to ensure the tree thrives. If we were to imagine a world that looks like that, that's held in interconnectedness, I feel like burnout would be so rare.'

Maymana pauses, and they inhale deeply before continu-ing excitedly – an example in real time of how our capacities for imagination expand when prompted to envisage them through hope. 'But wait, if we're saying that for burnout to be eradicated we must be resourced, then what would a post-burnout world look like? Because we'd have all our basic needs met, our planet's needs would also be met, and we wouldn't be scrambling to survive, we'd be living in a state of actual abundance. And I like the idea of that new state of being, where we're no longer having to unlearn capitalism, but instead are in a natural state of reciprocity, where we're all living through our relationships with one another, with the earth, the planet, with fungi, with plants, with all the living and non-living. It's nice to be reminded that that's what we're really working towards.'

It was this which we hoped to emulate during our walkshop. After lunch, we diverted from the footpath and nestled in a clearing surrounded by oak, elm and chestnut trees. In this private hideaway Bryony introduced us to a series of wild-drawing practices, each one encouraging us to blur the lines between the human and more-than-human. As we emerged from our ecological exhibition inky and muddy, with self-portraits, collaborative mycelium networks, detailed diagrams and line drawings under our arms, I found myself having to blink myself back to the present. I had been entirely lost to the world we had created here – present, yet far removed from the external realities. This felt surreal, given that we had travelled no distance at all, less than half a mile into the woodland in fact. We were no more than a ten-minute walk from the main road, and a fifteen-minute drive back to my own house, and yet I felt completely transported.

The entanglement with the earth that we had experienced here offered a taste of how our localised utopias could be realised and that it's possible to reimagine ourselves in the wider ecological networks from which we were once alienated. Ending our collaborative series with the Right to Roam campaign in this way somehow felt more like an opening. We began this journey in acknowledgement of the ways our grief and disconnect from the land are mutually destructive, explored how building an embodied practice which challenges the notion that our needs are separate to those of the environment, discarded all of the conditionings of white supremacy, and burrowed ourselves in and among fungi. A return to the earth, and the start of a new relationship with the land.

Hope, as a Black Feminist, Afrofuturist and abolitionist practice, redefines that which we can name and claim for ourselves. Within the foundations in which our revolutionary longings are cemented is a realisation: through a deeper connection to nature, each other and work that is grounded in a principle of experimentation, we can find hope that transcends the potential of burnout. We believe this is possible because we know that hope is solidified with the evidence of tangible action, creative imagination and community participation. It can be found in the infrastructures we build together, the mind-expansive moments we share together, the experiences in nature that replenish us and the comfort of knowing that, deep beneath our feet, there are the millions of fungal networks exhibiting connection and care.

Case Study #4: The Health Sector

*The history of illness has never just been plagues and the
invention of penicillin. It is a history of disparate access
to care. It is a history of devastation, a history of violence
via colonial experimentation and the organisation of
societies that continue to infect us. When we say this world
makes us sick, we mean that it is organised by capitalist
logics that produce precarity, instability of relation and
unlivable conditions. We mean that the big polluters give
us cancer, the carceral state sections us, pharmaceutical
companies drive up the price of life-saving drugs. The
state abandons us when the virus begins to circulate.*

*We say fuck the medical model and the algorithmic
diagnostics it uses to pathologise us. Our bodies are not the
problem. By poking holes in the medical model we propose
a methodology for being sick and keeping each other alive.*
 – Bare Minimum Collective.[1]

Given the detrimental impact of burnout on our physical
and emotional wellbeing, it may feel instinctive to look to
our current model of healthcare for direction. Understood
as being a form of 'socialised medicine', whereby the state
distributes healthcare to its citizens, the UK's NHS is considered a system to aspire to on the international stage.
Yet although the NHS may be comparatively more equitable than, for example, the US system, it is increasingly a

site of extreme neglect and harm and should, therefore, be interrogated.

Recent years in particular have seen the function of the NHS become warped amid rising privatisation. Access to care is increasingly being distributed in accordance with a social hierarchy, with those considered 'other' systematically denied care. That the maternal mortality rate of Black women is almost four times higher than of white women evidences this. As does the disproportionate rise in suicidality among trans young people caused by the state-sanctioned barriers to gender-affirming care,[2] and the inhumane conditions migrants must navigate if seeking support.

The authors of *Health Communism*, Beatrice Alder-Bolton and Artie Vierkant, pose that 'no such system of truly socialised medicine exists, or can exist, within the capitalist state.'[3] It's here that we can begin to understand that our considerations of burnout cannot rely on a healthcare system that actively contributes to the harm, and prevents the healing, of already vulnerable populations.

Health as State Suppression

Doctor, researcher and community organiser advocating for public health abolition, Kavian Kulasabanathan explains that: 'Capitalism makes us sick by turning us into a resource to be extracted. It's not just the extraction of labour, though that plays a big role. Capitalism also extracts our worth, energy and time. Time is such a finite resource yet capitalism steals our healthy years – time that should be dedicated to things that nourish us and bring us joy – in service of growth and greed.' Kavian organises with Race & Health and the People's Health Movement, two interdisciplinary networks committed to addressing the intersections of race and health injustice. Currently researching whether the state can ever truly provide health for all, Kavian joins me on Zoom from the UCL campus, squeezing me in between a protest in central London and his studies.

'Capitalism also makes us sick by denying us the basic things we need to survive: food, housing, heat, pleasurable activities. These structural oppressions – racism, trans-phobia, ableism, homophobia, misogyny – they show up in the body,' he continues. 'Then, it blames us for our inability to stay well, or get better, despite these horrific conditions. This sets unbelievably narrow terms around what it means to be healthy; able-bodied, mentally resilient, economic-ally privileged. Our health is measured against our ability to be a productive worker in aid of capital accumulation.'

We are currently seeing the devastating impacts of this across the UK. People who live in the poorest local authorities in Britain, including Sheffield and its neigh-bouring four towns in South Yorkshire, are 'vastly more likely' to live with poor health, be economically inac-tive and have some of the lowest life expectancy rates. In Barnsley for example, this is a shocking 61.5 years for women, and 57.5 years for men.[4] Azekel Axelle's story evi-dences this impact also. Azekel is the co-founder of the Black Trans Foundation, a non-profit organisation helping Black, trans and gender non-conforming people to access free and culturally safe healthcare. Founded in 2020, the Black Trans Foundation supported over fifty Black trans people in crisis within their first eighteen months of operations. A few years since its launch, however, Azekel and co-founder Jolliff are now in crisis themselves. Appealing for financial, emotional and advocacy support, through a GoFundMe page, the duo took to social media to ask for help, describing an 'unprecedented health crisis and severe mental and physical disability' as a result of 'burnout and overwork'. Organising on the front lines of a healthcare system that refuses to create space for the existence of Black trans people has ultimately been both life-altering and life-threatening for the team behind the Black Trans Foundation, and as a result, they have both lost the ability to walk.

Despite having followed their story on social media, I first met Azekel at a retreat for BIPOC activists, hosted by Decolonising Economics. We bonded quickly over our love for swimming and spent gleeful moments pretending to be merpeople in Welsh waters. Later that summer, I went to their house in Leeds to interview them. What followed was a wholesome day. Azekel had a membership to a nearby hotel's wellbeing facilities, which had a swimming pool, sauna and steam room. As we swam laps of the pool, we spent much of the afternoon talking through the intricacies of living with a disability – PIP forms, navigating the DWP and how much calmer, and in less pain, we respectively felt thanks to being in the water. When we returned to Azekel's shared flat, I warmed up some of their meal-prepped items that a carer prepares for them in the microwave and we ate together. When we commenced the interview, it was with me perched on a chair at the foot of the bed, and Azekel cosied up under the covers. I asked Azekel if they could paint a picture of their burnout journey, and the ways it has impacted their physical and mental health.

'When I started the Black Trans Foundation, I had some joint issues, a bit of pain here and there, but with painkillers it was manageable. It never stopped me from accessing society. By 2020, however, I was wearing knee supports daily, but still, just the ones you get from a shop. By 2021, I was wearing metal ones every day to walk, then had to upgrade to a splint alongside this. I was in extreme pain, but I was in such denial because – and it's embarrassing to admit – I was terrified of being disabled. This society teaches us that disability is not sexy, and naïvely I thought, 'I'm already dealing with being Black, and being trans, but having been socialised as a woman.' I felt I couldn't cope with a disability too.'

They tell me of how in the summer of 2022 there came a point where they stopped being able to walk for a week. The severity of their condition was at this point undeniable. 'I'd gone to a festival in London, navigated the pain as best as possible, and drank through the depression, then went home and found I couldn't get out of bed, not even to go to the toilet. My joints in my knees and my ankles felt like they were on fire. It was relentless. And I realised, there was no turning back at this point. I got my wheelchair that summer, but I now realise I'd been needing it for years,' they say, staring out of the window as they talk.

'Now we're looking at over a year's worth of just complete bodily degeneration. I was bed-bound for most of winter. I need care, *so* much care, but can't afford it. I need help going to the bathroom. I can't leave the house without assistance. The pain is unbearable, and I have chronic fatigue, depression and anxiety. Burnout *disables* people. The background stress of trying to meet your own basic needs, of dealing with racism and homophobia, and transphobia, *disables* people. And when you can't afford to be burnt out, you pay the price and then some.'

Throughout the day, I had assumed the role of carer for Azekel, and I was happy to help. At the Decolonising Economics retreat, Azekel's friend had been their main support, meaning I wasn't aware of the intricacies of their needs until invited to spend the day with them. Azekel has since moved back in with their mum so that their care needs could more readily be accessed, but at the time of my visit Azekel lived in a ground floor flat, accessed via a tiered ramp from the pavement to the front door. However, the three steps along this ramp meant that the flat wasn't accessible and their wheelchair had to live in the car, which was broken down on double yellow lines outside the flat. Azekel had to use a cane when both at home and when leaving the house which caused them immense pain and fatigue, and when we got to the car, the wheelchair was so heavy that it required two people to transfer it from their boot to mine. Without constant support, Azekel tells me, it's impossible for them to meet their own basic needs.

I asked if they could talk me through how their work with the Black Trans Foundation influenced their current condition. 'So, it was the height of the pandemic, and the Black Lives Matter movement was at its peak. I'd just managed to fundraise for my top surgery and was feeling overwhelmed by the racial trauma, and the communal feelings of rage we were surrounded by in the UK at the time. I wanted to be able to support Black trans people like me to access therapy sessions so that we could process what was happening around us. I applied for a grant that was designed to fund young people's ideas, and was successful. It was more money than I'd ever had for projects, but they said we weren't allowed to spend it on our wages because they just wanted to see 'community impact'. So we then had to fundraise for that. We managed to raise enough money to pay the wages of three people in our team, and I was so excited, but in hindsight what we were paying ourselves was so below minimum wage for the amount of work we were doing. I look back now and think, no wonder we burnt out.'

We talked of how as an employee in an average job you are often hired to do one particular role, which oversees a selection of tasks. As a founder, however, you find yourself doing every role in the organisation: creative director, admin manager, finance department, recruitment officer, fundraiser, community outreach officer, the list goes on. Yet it may be years of gruelling funding bids before you ever see yourself getting sufficiently paid, or being able to pay someone else to share some of the weight.

Azekel reels off a list of responsibilities they assumed in those early days of the Black Trans Foundation: 'I was recruiting and managing a team, overseeing twenty to thirty clients, sourcing organisational insurance, creating safeguarding policies, recording invoices, recruiting and interviewing therapists by scouring therapist directories (that only filter by race or sexuality, not both) for Black trans therapists, making application forms, hosting team meetings, partnering with other organisations, creating invoice templates, therapist profiles and a therapist directory on our website, registering as a community interest company, then dealing with all the horrific tax admin that comes with that, and being threatened with legal action by Companies House for getting it wrong.' They pause for breath before continuing. 'I ended up representing an entire department and doing five people's jobs at once. We ended up building a whole therapist organisation from the ground up, working with fifteen Black, trans or queer therapists, raised upwards of £100,000, distributed therapy to our community, supported student therapists, all while putting my university degree on hold I should add. At first it felt incredible, but it also became my identity. And it was towards the end of 2021 when I really started to feel like this work wasn't enjoyable any more. It felt like a huge responsibility, and I realised that as organisers, the team and I weren't looking after ourselves. My body just sort of fell apart.'

As Azekel's health was deteriorating, however, so was Jolliff's – their friend and Fundraising Manager at the Black Trans Foundation. Throughout their work together, both Azekel and Jolliff found their respective neurodivergencies contributed to the load of managing and running an organisation. The physical disabilities that developed however, compounded this, and it became clear that operating as 'business as usual' was not only impossible but irresponsible. As a result, the Black Trans Foundation, an organisation that became a lifeline for a community of people who are unable to access the same level of support through mainstream healthcare, have now paused their organising while their own recovery rightfully takes priority. Azekel tells me that the message they want to convey in this interview is both the severity of their condition as a cautionary tale, and of the ways that a non-disabled person can be disablised at any moment by the conditions under which the state forces us to work. 'If you don't rest, your body will make you rest,' they say.

Speaking to Azekel reiterates the importance of centring disability justice not only in our work, but in every facet of society. The work of Sins Invalid, a US-based project led by disabled people of colour committed to social and economic justice for people with disabilities, also reminds me of this. Their '10 principles of Disability Justice', which was created in 2015, has since been considered a fundamental tool in grassroots movement work worldwide. It includes: intersectionality, leadership of the most impacted, anti-capitalist politic, commitment to cross-movement organising, recognising wholeness, sustainability, commitment to cross-disability solidarity, interdependence, collective access and, ultimately, collective liberation. Considering such principles as fundamental to a healed and whole existence illuminates just how absent they are from the state's approach to ill health.

Under the medical model which both Azekel and Kavian describe, health becomes an unattainable fallacy, and those of us who are unable to medicate or 'self-care' ourselves into productivity are then rendered surplus. Though this surplus population constitutes a 'broad array of categorisations and are united in their degrees of being, for one reason or another, certified biologically, socially and politically as surplus', Adler-Bolton and Vierkant explain that 'once certified as surplus, these populations are then used to stave off broad reforms that would otherwise be destabilising to capitalism, usually through an argument that the surplus constitutes a burden to society in two ways: first as a eugenic burden, then as a debt burden'.[5]

Through this lens we can see how, together, the workplace, welfare state and healthcare perpetrate a slow and bureaucratic violence against those considered surplus. Those of us who are disabled or chronically ill are discarded by the state, then penalised through the benefits system – in which 93 per cent of people say the process of claiming benefits makes their mental health worse, and 61 per cent say the system has caused them to have suicidal thoughts, with 13 per cent attempting suicide as a result of interacting with the DWP. How can we look to the state for any kind of support in our burnout recovery when there is such potential for further harm? This multifaceted approach to institutional alienation, which ensures the precarity and vulnerability of surplus populations by denying and manipulating resources, is what Ruth Wilson Gilmore describes as 'organised abandonment'.[6]

Health as Racial (In)Justice

The current conditions of our medical systems are not a new phenomenon. They in fact represent the enduring legacy of medical racism, which still informs much of our experience of neglect and suffering within present-day healthcare. As the doctor, activist and academic Dr Annabel Sowemimo explains, 'Some of the earliest European colonial explorers in the sixteenth century turned to science to justify their own prejudicial beliefs on white, European superiority.'[7] In *Divided: Racism, Medicine and Why We Need to Decolonise Healthcare*, she points to some of the British and European colonial physicians and academics who, during the height of the British Empire, established the notion that race was integral to understanding disease.

Darwin was among those credited, with his theory of natural selection acting in many ways as the catalyst for the eugenics movement which followed. Drawing on the Greek word *eugenes*, meaning 'good in stock, hereditarily endowed with noble qualities', eugenics' preoccupation with the betterment of the human species was reliant on maintaining white racial superiority,[8] inspiring many of the practices that went on to become central to some of the Nazis' experiments as they looked to justify a racial hierarchy during the Holocaust.

Sowemimo highlights how, despite race science evolving throughout history, its existence 'would provide a "scientific" reason for the ongoing subjugation of those deemed physically and mentally inferior.'[9] Race science was used to maintain slavery, expand overseas colonies and implement segregation, and we can see this still being reapplied today: within right-wing rhetoric, to dehumanise immigrants and Palestinians, at the core of fascist feminist calls to suppress access to gender-affirming healthcare, and in the justification of scaled policing against Black communities.

This is something that Micha Frazer-Carroll highlights throughout *Mad World: The Politics of Mental Health*. She finds that rather than care, it is a desire to deny Black people's ability to organise and mobilise against systemic racism which often informs psychiatric diagnoses.

'Drapetomania', for example, was a diagnosis given to Black enslaved people who fled plantations, deeming their desire for freedom a cognitive impairment. Meanwhile, the diagnosis we recognise today as schizophrenia has gone through many iterations of weaponisation. In the 1960s, for example, it was dubbed 'the protest psychosis', a frequent diagnosis assigned to civil rights organisers, as a way of dismissing their legitimate distress at and resistance to inequality.

Today, mental health conditions considered the most severe continue to be disproportionately diagnosed in racialised communities. Black men are ten times more likely to receive a diagnosis of a psychotic disorder than their white counterparts,[10] while Black Caribbean people are nine times more likely to receive a schizophrenia diagnosis.[11] 'Notably, this extremely high rate of diagnosis in the UK has not been replicated in the Caribbean,' Micha points out, highlighting the somewhat contradictory ways that Black people's legitimate trauma is both ignored and exacerbated. 'Since the experiences described as schizophrenia are often thought to be linked to stress and trauma, these rates of diagnosis might be considered entirely representative of our lived realities [...] Living in contemporary Britain continues to be traumatising for many people of colour – with racism embedded in each of its institutions.'[12]

History, and indeed the ongoing present, teaches us that we cannot trust the state to provide support in our burnout recovery. Though a disability justice lens may support us to understand our experiences of burnout as something that is disabling, impairing, sickening, maddening and chronic, we must proceed with caution before inviting the state to also pathologise us as such. While an institutional awareness of burnout could offer the opportunity for some to be taken more seriously in their suffering, it also risks endangering Black, queer, disabled people of colour – particularly those who participate in movement work – further. By rendering us surplus, it may also be the catalyst for the kinds of further state-surveillance and oppression we have seen elsewhere – institutionalisation, denied citizenship, criminalisation or the removal of children.

Health as an Industrial Complex

That so many of the medical interventions available to us result in increased incarceration, as opposed to increased care, is no accident. As Angela Davis elaborates in *Are Prisons Obsolete?*, healthcare as we know it is a functioning cog within a carceral system. The distribution of so-called psychiatric support is an example of this. 'While jails and prisons have been dominant institutions for the control of men, mental institutions have served a similar purpose for women,' she writes. 'That deviant men have been constructed as criminal, while deviant women have been constructed as insane'[13] supports an understanding that healthcare has intentionally become an extension of the prison industrial complex.

In the UK, policing disguised as care is enshrined in law. Section 136 of The Mental Health Act 1983, for example, sanctions carceral methods of violence by giving the police the power to search and detain any person they believe to have a mental illness. Blurring the lines between support and criminalisation further, it's likely that once a person has been detained they will find themselves in a psychiatric institution. Much like a prison, these so-called 'care' facilities now routinely have police situated within them, and treatment is often distributed through coercion and lack of consent.

Resisting the notion that psychiatry is a benevolent and caring institution, and raising awareness of the historic and contemporary atrocities committed by those under the guise of 'mental health care', Campaign for Psychiatric Abolition is a group comprised of psychiatric survivors – or, as their Twitter bio describes themselves, 'fuckin lunatics' – who emerged in the UK in 2021. CPA's three-point strategy includes political education, mutual aid and direct action. The latter is achieved through the organisation of Mad Pride, an action which carries the legacy of a long history of survivor-led anti-psychiatry resistance in the UK and beyond.

With placards brandishing slogans such as 'Fuck the Mind Police', 'Disordered and ready to organise' and 'Maybe it's the world that's Mad', CPA's 2021 march led a psychiatric abolition resurgence. The parade offered a new generation of survivors a political platform on which to make visible the institutional violence that often goes unnoticed. It also honoured traditional actions such as the 'bed push' – something of a performance piece, aided with props like a giant syringe, that depicts a person or dummy being liberated from the psych ward by being pushed on a hospital bed, through the streets, to freedom.

Though it is understood that so many of us must continue to navigate and interact with the current systems of healthcare in order to receive some semblance of support, the campaign rejects the presence of such institutions at the front lines. Ahead of the protest, they issued a statement saying: 'Just as we wouldn't let cops in police abolitionist spaces, or prison officers in prison abolitionist spaces, there is no place for mental health "professionals" of ANY kind in psychiatric abolitionist spaces.'[14] Citing the ways such professionals have traumatised so many of the organisers, how it would be impossible to celebrate madness among those who routinely try to suppress and erase it, and of the ways that including professionals in said spaces routinely de-radicalises and removes safety from the space, CPA speak to the ways that active complicity is built into job roles deemed to be 'caring'.

This is a complicity that Kavian and I have both negotiated: me as a domestic abuse and psychiatric survivor working within the VAWG sector, and Kavian as a medical practitioner. When I ask Kavian how he navigates these tensions, he tells me: 'I've found it really hard, unsurprisingly. There's punitive systems that are explicitly control-oriented. Arms of the state like border control, the police force, and we're told there's a distinction between these and the more traditional, care-oriented arms of the state, like healthcare, social care, schools. But in reality these sides have collapsed in on each other.' As an example, we discuss how PREVENT – a so-called anti-terrorist scheme whereby the government enlists local authorities and community organisations to racially profile and police their service users – is embedded into standard practice within both the health and the VAWG sector, and how practitioners are penalised for their non-compliance.

'We live within, and are attempting to reimagine within, the structures that we're critiquing,' Kavian says.

Health as Healing Justice

The state's inaction around burnout, and how it suspends us between 'worker' and 'surplus' with perverse subtlety, can be understood as organised abandonment. Although it is the pressure of the capitalist system that has rendered us 'unfit' to work, and though plenty of research supports the classification of burnout as a chronic illness, burnout is still considered akin to stress in much public and institutional rhetoric. Though we don't advocate for pathologisation here, in our current system this has significant repercussions when it comes to access to benefits, reasonable adjustments or medical support. As an arbitrary measure of who is deserving or undeserving of care, a diagnosable, institutionally recognised condition is often required. This means that even the state-sanctioned forms of patienthood, no matter how deplorable, are unavailable to us, the burnt out.

What this presents, however, is an opportunity, and through grassroots organising we see that rather than striving for inclusion in a system that ultimately will never care about us, it is our collective solidarity that will suture capitalism's gaping wounds. Given the risks that pathologisation and institutionalisation pose, perhaps this is an opportunity, an opening. Perhaps we can build a liberatory form of healthcare system which is life-affirming and dignifying. One which centres people who capitalism would consider surplus, so that we might – as Gilmore describes – 'organise against our abandonment.'[15] A healthcare

system in which, instead of abandonment, we are prescribed community. Instead of pathologisation, we are
prescribed healing. Instead of institutionalisation, we
are prescribed justice. Instead of capitalism, we are
prescribed revolution.

On Radical Rest

And, oh God, let's all have a capacity to feel. Let our
work be towards expanding our capacity of feeling.
— Elizabeth-Jane Burnett[1]

W hen we began this journey together, Octavia E. Butler's
novel *Parable of the Sower* and the diaries of her main
protagonist, Lauren, grounded our introduction to burnout in a
speculative present-future. In Lauren's final journal entries, she
details the hopeful possibility of a new beginning for herself
and the trusting disciples she has gathered along the perilous
journey to safety. It's 2027 now, and after an arduous expedition
across the USA on foot, they find a plot of land that her partner,
Bankhole, owns 'free and clear'. Surrounded by pine trees and
redwoods, the land is hidden away from the atrocities of contemporary America. It has plots for farming, for building, an orchard
full of fruit and nut trees. 'It will be hard to live here, but if
we work together, and if we're careful, it should be possible,'[2]
Lauren writes.

Lauren is viscerally conscious of the ways that the stewardship
of this land is integral to her sprouting community's autonomy. It
will enable them to be self-sufficient and self-determining as they
build a sanctuary that is safe from the ills of the sick society outside. Yet — as we have come to understand in our excavation of our
emotions in previous chapters — these weary refugees have matters
of the mind, body and soul to tend to first. They hold ceremonies

for their dead, for those they had to flee and for the former selves they also lost along the way. Only after this meditative naming and letting-go of the traumas they carried, and a commitment to continual healing, can the rebuilding begin. And rebuild they do. They name their community Earthseed and through a thriving commitment to care, they begin planning for the world they want, transforming this land into a place of respite. As we too look towards a present-future in which rest – and a burnout-free existence – feels possible, it is a rooting in justice, dreaming and place that we explore in this, our concluding chapter.

Rest as Land Justice

Since I began writing *Radical Rest*, the collapse of civilisation as we know it has begun to unfold. Though it may not have yet reached Western shores, the ongoing genocidal campaign against Palestine – which is said to claim an estimated 250 lives a day, more than any other twenty-first-century conflict[3] – can, in many ways, be seen as a realisation of Butler's apocalyptic premonition. This has been the first genocide where so much of the inhumanity has been captured live, and as we bear witness to the moral atrocities, those of us in the West have received a humbling education in the façade of so-called democracy and international human rights law, the abject cruelty that our Western governments are capable of endorsing, and, in contrast, of the power of individual action and the strength of a global collective resistance.

One overwhelming lesson, however, is the undeniable ways that land justice, racial justice and health justice intersect. Prior to the most recent developments in this ongoing occupation, Palestinians cultivated an abundant variety of crops, but the bulldozing of agricultural lands, combined with the historic spraying of herbicides and the restriction and pollution of groundwater has led to the destruction of former arable land.[4] This renders communities destitute and severs Palestinians from the rich tradition of farming and agriculture. Coupled with the restriction of humanitarian aid, the malnutrition and starvation of a people is not only orchestrated in the present, but the possibility of rebuilding remains untenable for future generations, due to the ecological disruption of the region's landscapes.

Political philosopher Frantz Fanon wrote: 'For a colonised people, the most essential value, because it is the most meaningful, is first and foremost the land: the land, which must provide bread and, naturally, dignity.'[5] Three images immediately spring to mind when considering how a tactic of settler colonialism is to target the environment, which then indirectly impacts the people. The first is a sepia photo of two white men that was taken in 1892. One stands atop a mountain of initially unidentifiable objects, which towers above the second man standing at its base. Both are proudly resting with one leg upon their trophies. To squint reveals that this manufactured landscape is in fact built of bones. This mountainous graveyard is constructed of buffalo skulls and represents how an animal considered an important economic, cultural and spiritual symbol among many indigenous nations was killed by settlers to starve Native Americans and force those who survived into reservations. An estimated 8 million bison roamed Turtle Island (the Indigenous nations' name for what is now the United States) at the time. But within just twenty years, they were on the brink of extinction, with fewer than 500 remaining. The economic, cultural and health repercussions of this targetisation have reverberated through indigenous communities ever since.

The second image, taken in 2005, is of a Palestinian woman embracing the trunk of an olive tree. With her eyes closed and mouth open in despair, the woman clutches the tree as Israeli soldiers loom in the background, the threat of fertile land stolen through military aggression imminent. Fifteen years later the farmer, Mahfodah Shtayyeh, spoke to Al Jazeera: 'I hugged the olive tree, it was precious to me, so I hugged it. I felt like I was hugging my child. I raised the tree like my child,' she tells the reporter. Since the Naksa (an exodus of hundreds of thousands of Palestinians, following the war and occupation in 1967), 80,000 olive trees stewarded by Palestinians in the occupied West Bank have been uprooted.[6] Olive trees – which alongside the watermelon have since become an emblem of Palestinian national identity, connection to homeland and resistance – are also a vital source of income. 'They destroyed my olive trees, but I grew them back. I tended to them, and they came back even better than before. Settlers will never be able to take my land, this is our land not theirs. We will keep resisting until the world ends,' Shtayyeh says.[7]

The final image speaks to how a spiritual love for and deep devotion to nature has the power to transcend violence. Taken in 2013 near the de facto Palestinian capital of Ramallah in the West Bank, the photograph, captured among a series of images, focuses upon another Palestinian woman, this time tending to her garden. At her feet lies a carpet of flowers planted in used tear gas grenades. Hundreds of these makeshift plant pots adorn a hillside contained by barbed wire fencing. Though it's a stark reminder of the violence used by Israel in an attempt to fracture the relationship with the land that Palestinians have nurtured over generations, close-ups of this woman's hands show the care applied to these bombs, as life in the form of green shoots and pink flowers bloom from the remnants of weaponised suffering.

When I think of the ways such nurturing has the power to grow beauty from the wreckage of harm, I think of Her Farm, a matriarchal, women-only community where I spent some time conducting research during my postgraduate degree in 2018. Founded by Sunita Subedi Sharma, a survivor of domestic abuse in an arranged marriage, Her Farm is based in the rural, mountainous hills of Nepal.[8] Taking the road that leads out of Katmandu to Pokhara, I arrived at Her Farm by bus, which dropped me off at a village where a small row of shops lines a dusty main road, like an old Western movie. From here I was picked up by one of the men who support the community, his car following a dirt path that winds around the hills like a helter-skelter. Finally, we arrived at the gates of a modest complex, tucked away in the mountain range.

What unites the women at Her Farm is their experience of fleeing patriarchal violence. Whether they have survived domestic abuse, sexual exploitation, forced marriage, institutional harm, community persecution or familial ostracisation, they all came to Her Farm in search of sanctuary and possibility. Any male relatives, including Sunita's own husband, live nearby. Inside the community, however, women and children exist in safety and solidarity.

One thing that struck me was the expansive approach to self-fulfilment that was practised here. Everyone had a role that they had chosen for themselves. These roles contributed to the functioning of the community, and yet offered exactly what each individual needed to feel content. Those interested in accessing an education were supported feverishly in their passions. A community health centre was erected for those who were training to be nurses, broadcast equipment was sourced for those interested in starting the first women-run community radio in the area, and donors were found to contribute state-of-the-art cameras to those who wanted to explore photography, for example. Many of the women were skilled in agriculture and their interests in environmental stewardship and sustainability were supported as they tended to the land. Meanwhile, those who were content looking after children or assuming responsibility for domestic duties, such as preparing meals, did so without any pressure to overachieve.

Similarly impressive were the ways the community transformed once-oppressive structures of colonial dominance to their own ends. Sunita's husband's Western connections were utilised to ensure that the community was resourced in state-of-the-art technology is one example. Western tourists and volunteers were hosted for a fee, and while they were given access to everyday amenities, they received none of the entitled rewards of voluntourism and white saviourism, other than being taught an important lesson: communities in so-called 'developing countries' don't actually need white saviours to rescue them.

I was in my early twenties, and still in an abusive relationship at the time of my visit. Her Farm was one of the first places I experienced the possibility of a life entirely autonomous from patriarchal racial capitalism. This wasn't something that could be dismissed as mere speculative fiction, but a real, undeniable haven for Nepalese women, where rest was synonymous with freedom from oppression, and made possible through land sovereignty. Though our request for rest may seem incomparable to the pleas for life in Palestine, what we can learn from Sunita's Her Farm, Lauren's Earthseed and Mahfodah's Palestine is that there are common prerequisites when acting on what we need to ensure our holistic healing. Space for dreaming, self-determination, freedom of creative expression, community care and collective responsibility, the opportunity to heal old wounds while divesting from all that could continue to harm, and . . . land.

Rest as a Dreamland

As Peaks of Colour continues its journey in earnest, I find myself in a constant self-dialogue around what our community's own place of radical rest could look and feel like. Returning to these aspirational requirements offers guidance on what this could be – a dreamhouse, a dreamscape, a dreamland – and how we could manifest it.

Throughout the *Parables* books, Lauren's hyper-empathy is constantly positioned as a disabling vulnerability, something to be ashamed of, to be hidden. In Peaks of Colour's dreamhouse, however, the depth of our emotions will be celebrated within the very walls, the very foundations of our home. We will enter and be enveloped in a cloud of care and healing, intimately designed through a desire to reach and massage the deepest knots of our traumas. Stewarded by an array of racial justice organisers, each room will be an embodied, experiential escape. Carefully curated to evoke or address an emotion, they will thereby transform our feelings and needs into strengths and solidarities, rather than weaknesses under a capitalist production. Of the emotions that we have explored in this book together, our exhaustion will signal our need for rest, a need to pause, to take stock, recuperate and slow down. Our anger will be honoured as the teacher of boundaries and will be released without fear or judgement. Our grief will be ritualised as the one true unifier, transformed into collective action in service of the memory of those who came before us. Our anxiety will be our compass as we search for the embodied evidence that guides us to move only through what feels good and sit with the discomfort of what doesn't.

Our needs – material, monetary, practical, physical and emotional – will be resourced, not least by the abundance of what the land can offer us, but also through a community library filled with books, tools and resources, an ancestral archive, and a drop-in space where people can be supported with life skills and admin, such as completing a PIP form, language exchange or political education. There will be rooms for residentials and rooms for vulnerable unhoused members of the community. There will be a free crèche for the young and care facilities for the elderly, and office and studio space allocated to each collaborator, so that we have space to strategise and commune.

Our joy will be an electric current that flows through our dreamland – a permanent feature of the work, not a fleeting moment amid overwhelming resilience. Alongside space for a multimedia arts studio, a sensory room, a playroom, a community radio and a cinema room, so that our everyday can be laced with joyful practice, there will be a dance hall that by day acts as a space for exhibitions and events, and by night is kitted out with the finest decks and karaoke sets. Here, our capacity to hope for and imagine a life-affirming present-future will expand to infinite lengths. And of course, there are other emotions that contribute to burnout which we haven't covered on this written journey together, such as fear, shame, guilt and envy. In our dreamhouse, we will have space and time to address these too. Trust, forgiveness, gratitude, love (of the self and of each other) can often feel scarce in our current movement spaces. In our dreamhouse they will be nurtured.

Surrounding our dreamhouse would be our dreamland. This land would be plentiful, and together we will build land-based skills of self-sufficiency. Our meadows will bloom wildflowers that nourish the bees and wildlife. We will tend to allotments and orchards that supply homegrown food to our community kitchen, while in our herbal garden we will populate medicines for an in-house apothecary. On farmland we'll care for an abundance of animal kin – the lifelong vegetarian-turned-vegan in me can't consent to them being eaten, I'm afraid – but through our tending to an array of creatures, we will develop a greater sense of responsibility and relationship. The land will be vast enough for us to disappear off into the hills on group excursions, but closer to home we will also have access to canopied therapeutic areas: pergolas and tree houses in which to host regular yoga, sound-bathing or meditation sessions, grief circles and ancestral ceremonies, individual and group therapies, and workshops around conflict resolution or abolitionist practice. And, of course, any dreamland in my imagination must include a vast body of water. A lake, a river or a waterfall trail, perhaps, where daily wild swims can refresh our nervous systems and connect us in embodied, nature-allied practice.

When I picture each room in this dreamhouse, and how they will be designed to facilitate a restful escape, Black Power Naps come to mind. Black Power Naps is an American-based interactive and artistic initiative curated by queer, Black Latinx American duo Navild Acosta and Fannie Sosa. Displayed at the MoMA in New York City throughout 2023, their exhibition invited audiences to experience a restful liberation, reclaiming laziness and idleness as a powerful force for reparations and repairs.

Featured in this installation was their 'Pelvic Floor', a trampoline surrounded by subwoofers acting as a membrane that amplified the vibration of muscles, proven to aid stress and trauma. A piece called 'Atlantic Reconciliation' paid homage to the Atlantic Ocean as a place where so many Black and indigenous ancestors were lost. Using bass frequencies, it aimed to rejuvenate the stagnant water that sits in our bodies, utilising water as a tool for rest. Their 'Poly-Crastination Station' was a comfortable surface on which to lie down, with a hanging vanity and mirror above it that invited participants to look inward and practice self-love, self-reflection and self-awareness. As Navild says, 'To look at your-self you gotta lay down, boo.'[9]

Another piece on offer was 'The Oxygenation Swing', a collection of draped and swaying hammocks. Here air currents were used to create better circulation, causing the resting body to breathe more deeply, leading to better quality sleep. And finally, there was the 'Black Bean Bed', which according to the pair has been popular with the senior population. It was designed with panic attacks in mind and includes a pool filled with two tonnes of dry black beans, heavy blankets and cushions with fresh herbs hanging above them.

The phenomenon of dreaming appears to be a universal feature of the human experience, yet research conducted during the Black Lives Matter uprising in the wake of George Floyd's murder considered the relationship between dreaming and race. Seeking to explore how our dreams are impacted during a time of heightened collective awareness, the study revealed that those most likely to have dreams of racial injustice were those who supported and were involved in Black Lives Matter. These dreams, the research found, tended to be anxious, fearful, nightmarish and centred around themes of threat and harm. 'I keep replaying the guy dying and saying, "I can't breathe, Momma,"' one person recalled, while another found they kept reliving the moment they were tear gassed during a protest.

Perhaps this is why 'political *unrest*' is called exactly that – not just to name the systemic ways in which it disrupts, but because it also confines those of us impacted and involved in movement work to a trauma response that replays our own suffering even in sleep. It's for this reason that carving out spaces for a restful imagination, spaces where we are permitted to dream beyond our current realities, is vital. In curating spaces out of everyday cultural items,

Black Power Naps showcase that we already possess the tools and materials needed for deep rest. That despite the multifaceted ways we are pushed towards burnout, when the imaginary possibilities of creative design are combined with ancestral wisdoms and cultural resources, the ability to dream of, then create, a haven for healing is already in our hands.

The sceptics will say that this dreamland is just that – a dream. To that I say, duh! The incremental freedoms that we have succeeded in actualising thus far have all been the product of our ancestors' dreams and fights for freedom. At one point in time, the abolition of slavery would have seemed as fanciful and idealistic as our calls for a free Palestine in our lifetime, the abolition of systems of policing that thrive under racial capitalism, or the eradication of burnout as the ongoing trauma of the present day.

In the face of so many assaults to our sense of self, the serene, regulated, peaceful state of rest emerges as an emotion we wish to nurture. Doing so not only offers the opportunity for us to dream beyond our present conditions, but gifts us with the replenished capacity needed for us to turn those dreams into a reality. And thus, the cycle begins: the more we rest, the more we dream. The more we dream, the more we divest and build. The more we divest and build, the more we rest.

The sceptics may also say there isn't enough land on which we can build our dreamhouse. To that I say: that simply isn't true. Anyone who has ever had a bird's eye view from the seat of an aeroplane of the patchwork quilt that is the UK landscape will know this too. Currently, half of England is owned by less than 1 per cent of the population and less than 1 per cent of the population residing in rural areas are from global majority communities.[10] But if the land were distributed evenly across England, it's estimated that each person would have just over half an acre.

The land exists, as do examples of land stewarded by communities of colour. In the Peak District, the Chatsworth Estate and Tissington Hall are still owned and lived in by the descendants of slave owners. These properties could be viable options for our dreams to manifest. Or perhaps we could steward Wentworth Castle, Kedleston Hall, Hardwick Hall and Calke Abbey, four properties around Derbyshire and South Yorkshire under the National Trust's management, revealed in their recent report as having direct links to slavery.[11] Maybe the royal family could give up some of their 287,000 acres of private land?[12] Or perhaps our home could be found elsewhere, somewhere untouched, unscathed. Somewhere that isn't haunted by the ghosts of a colonial past. If such a place exists.

Black Power Naps' mission statement reads: 'As Afro Latinx artists, we believe that reparation must come from the institution under many shapes, one of them being the redistribution of rest, relaxation, and down times.' There is a recognition here that though we, as racialised communities, may commit the time and energy required to transform our deepest emotions and our long-standing traumas into something regenerative, our rest can only be truly sustained with our complete liberation. This requires those benefiting from power and privilege under the dominant system of racial capitalism to open themselves up to the unlearning and sacrifices required for a revolution such as this. 'To centre the [rest] of Black folk, you must not economise, commodify or extort it: hand over the keys and leadership, allow the experts to guide,' Black Power Naps advocate. 'Let the ask include energetic reparations in the form of access to healthy sustainable and rejuvenating leisure rest and quality sleep.'[13]

I'm not naïve to the fact that to actualise this dreamland in this economic and political climate will be difficult, but as long as we are forced to do the work of healing, of resting, of dreaming within the walls of white supremacy, we will only ever be halfway there. This dream will take time, energy, people power, our wildest imaginations, and the financial and land reparations of the privileged. Maybe a dream is all that it is right now, but this vision for our collective future wasn't even a glimmer in my mind a year ago. Back then, I was merely dreaming of not suffering in this work, and yet I currently feel a sense of hopeful openness similar to Lauren's in *Parables*. 'I may not know how to build it [...] but I'm just feeling my way, using whatever I can do, whatever I can learn to take one more step forward!' she writes.[14]

Radical Rest

When I initially introduced my understanding of burnout, I wrote that the solutions are not quick or easy fixes. Somehow this truth feels more disappointing and insufficient now, when we've made our way through each of these emotion-centred chapters, than it did at the start. Knowing how much self-work and collective work must go into actualising radical rest can be an overwhelmingly daunting foresight to possess. Yet, one of Lauren's parables reads: 'Nothing eases the pain except rest [...] We're all sore and sick, in mourning and exhausted [...] we are a harvest of survivors. But then, that's what we've always been',[15] and suddenly we are reminded that even the darkest corners of our traumas hold the potential for strength, for transformation.

What this ongoing burnout recovery journey has taught me is that this resistance will require a conscious effort, as healing does for so many of us already. That routinely unlearning the conditions of racial capitalism will feel as uncomfortable and as unnatural as a detox: vulnerable, overwhelming and anticipatory. But it's also taught me that in the excavation of our feelings lies the opportunity for rebirth; that it is in our collective love for ourselves, each other and the earth that we will discover the possibilities for a restful revolution; and that in the mutual reciprocity of dreamlands such as those I have conjured here, it is possible for our understanding of rest to transcend something radical, becoming simply a normalised feature of our existence. Here we can harness the belief that burnout can be eradicated.

This book has borne witness to this journey. Throughout the writing process I've continued to grapple with my place in the movement. I've traversed the peaks and troughs of belonging, the highs of hopeful purpose, self-discovery, successful funding bids, emotive moments of connection, hopeful dreaming. And the lows of traumatic relapse, institutional fuckery, unsuccessful funding bids, instinctive overextending, and a premature opening of old, old wounds. I've burnt out numerous times despite my best efforts, but also looked for learnings and openings in these moments and emerged with a gradually evolving trust in my ability to persevere – to live. Despite being consistently overwhelmed by my emotional response to ongoing harm, I have noticed that the day-to-day centring of rest over production has begun to feel more like an instinct. Though the emergence of a future healed version of myself is contingent on the emergence of a healed society, at times this feels tantalisingly within reach. And it could be so – should be so – for all of us.

Much like Peaks of Colour's walkshops, *Radical Rest* has been a journey of exploration that I knew I couldn't do alone. Every facet of my work is done in and with community and, though it has necessitated lonesome moments of personal introspection, this book has been no different. Angela Davis reminds us that 'anybody who is interested in making change in this world, also has to learn how to take care of himself, herself, themselves',[16] and it is for this reason that the words, thoughts, wisdoms, musings, reflections and assertions of almost twenty people whose work dares to dream of a transformed future sit on these pages. These are Black and people of colour, most of whom are queer and/or disabled, many of whom are trans, gender-non-conforming, neurodivergent, all of whom are reckoning with their own experiences of burnout. And all are feverishly dedicated to overthrowing the oppressive, exploitative, stifling, exhausting, traumatising structures that cause our emotional exhaustion.

This will not be a singular event. This revolution demands of us a commitment to everyday acts of abolition as the 'ongoing process of assessing and replacing any system that doesn't serve all of us':[17] the massaging of the muscle that is our radical imagination; the prioritisation of care and love in the face of abject hatred and abandonment; the healing of the traumas inflicted on us by systems of harm; the challenging of carceral and punitive conditions which keep us disassociated and disembodied; and the building of collective capacity for safety, healing and connection as a tool of prevention and repair. These are not small implementations, granted. A plaster will never suffice to heal the seeping intergenerational wounds of our collective traumas, and we must reckon with the inconvenient truth that we may never be able to experience unconditional rest under racial capitalism in this lifetime. But, together, we share a collective understanding – that only by facilitating such societal collapse can we build an alternative abolitionist future where we can truly, truly rest.

Yet, activist burnout comes from the expectation that a few people should shoulder the responsibility of saving, fixing, holding, fighting. It is here we extend the invitation and ask others to join us in this care-full, rest-full resistance. The future we are envisioning is not one where traumatised and broken individuals reinvent a traumatising and breakable society. It is one where a healed, whole, hopeful coalition build a healed, whole, hopeful alternative. Our ability to look after ourselves must never come at the expense of another's time or labour. Rather, our ability to heal is dependent upon the involvement of *everyone*. When we speak of rest in this way, we do not advocate for something idle, luxurious, individualistic or indulgent. This is not a reminder to those sitting in their ivory towers to book that spa day. It is a call to arms, a desperate cry for help, a demand for you to join us in this fight. When creating a society in which burnout no longer exists, we all have a role to play, a skill to utilise, a resource to share in beginning to incorporate restful, hopeful, joyful and loving practices *right now*.

When people ask me where I see Peaks of Colour in X years' time, my answer is usually, *I don't know, and that's okay*. As our work grows and deepens, however, I am beginning to understand our role in this movement to be one of capacity-building for the revolution that must follow. One that creates spaces that tend to the parts of us which, under normal circumstances, would be suppressed, ignored and forgotten – the grief, the sorrow, the heartache, the anger, the pain, the anxiety, the fear, the shame. All that which inconveniences racial capitalism. All that is left to fester and corrode, ignite and, eventually, burn out.

Our role is to hold space where time is suspended, elongated. An elastic, transcendent sense of being exactly where we need to be. Through the creation of spaces where radical tenderness is centred, we are permitted to submit to the rest that our bodies ache for. The fleshy terrains of resistance which we inhabit hold all that hurts – our role must be to facilitate an evolution of self that transforms our darkest, most destructive of emotions into postures where freedom is felt.

Our role is to create spaces of togetherness. When capitalism wants us to remain isolated and alone, depending upon its manufactured, consumerist, piecemeal crumbs of connection, we say no. Let's repair the ties that have been severed, remedy the wounds that keep us separated, and rebuild a thriving, loving home for ourselves, on our terms. The strength of this connection ensures that not one of us feels alone in this struggle, in this recovery or in this fight. When united within an ecosystem of care, we're not only nurturing resilient individuals but a resilient collective. An impenetrable fortress. And in doing so, the embers of our movement are not extinguished simply because one of us must rest. When one must pause, others step in, and the momentum remains. We can't heal from burnout in isolation, and so, an embodied and trauma-informed recovery, held in the warm embrace of community care, is non-negotiable.

Our role is also to ensure that this journey is nature-allied. My own exploration has been so intimately enmeshed with my love for and dependency on nature as a tool for healing that it would be impossible to untangle it, even if I wanted to. Nature is fundamental to our healing from burnout — and our oppressors, past and present, recognise this. Their attempts to separate and isolate us from the land expose a conscious understanding of our human and more-than-human dependencies — that the destruction of natural resources facilitates the destruction of a life emboldened with agency, dignity, joy, hope and rest. Across the world, throughout the ongoing resistance to a colonial power, indigenous peoples' unwavering love for their land has been a constant reminder of our ecological accountabilities. An honouring of the enduring struggles for land justice is therefore what we must strive to mirror in our decolonial ethic. We must ask:

Who do we become when we understand that our oppression is inseparable from the exploitation of the land, and that our liberation is dependent upon an ecological freedom?

Who do we become when permitted to feel our aliveness in all its raw imperfections?

Who do we become when we build homes of togetherness in the tactile landscapes of our emotions?

Who do we become when we let our burnout, and our insatiable need for rest, radicalise us?

Holding these questions – suspending them in mid-air for us to examine, ponder over, witness, tend to and immerse ourselves in – is also what I understand our role to be. Creating capacity for hope, for possibility, for visioning, imagining, weaving, for otherwise and elsewhere, for who-knows and what-ifs. For an excitable trust in the process. An inquisitive exploration of the unknown. An expansive curiosity. An unquantifiable knowing that freedom is possible. We are our own experiment. We are our own evidence. This is radical rest. It is destructive work. It is worldbuilding work. It is communal work. It is dreaming work. It is future work. It is imaginative work. It is vulnerable work. It is feeling work. It is natured work. It is hopeful work. It is excavating work. It is liberating work. And, I believe, it is entirely possible.

Glossary of Re-definitions

Redefining 'Burnout' through a Lived
Experience of Racial (In)Justice

Writer and poet Toni Morrison said: 'Definitions belong to the definers, not the defined.'[1] As we have come to understand throughout *Radical Rest*, the current understanding of burnout is woefully inadequate and fails to capture the intricacies of an intersectional lived experience. During the research process, I asked each of the interviewees featured in this book to describe or define burnout, through a personal or political lens. In this, our Glossary of Re-definitions, we excavate honesty and reclaim our truth.

'This idea of "Zombie Time" really resonated with so many of us in the collective. Those of us who understand ourselves as in a state between life, and living, and some form of social, spiritual death. I think burnout can be put in that category, along that continuum. Framed this way when people describe capitalism as a "death machine", burnout allows us to understand it more as a machine that keeps us just alive enough to stay in or go back to work. And because what we need for living is made into profit, we all exist in conditions that drive us to this place of burnout.'

— *Vera Chapiro (Bare Minimum Collective)*

'The thing that leaps out to me about burnout is that it's the individual impact of a process that extracts lifeforce from people in service of capital. It makes me think of in particular the racialised working class, who are conceptualised as a resource and extracted from, then tossed aside, like a fossil fuel, or like wood from a forest. Burnout is the process of essentially being burned, finished, and then discarded in service of the accumulation of capital.'

– Kavian Kulasabanathan (Race and Health)

'I often see my existence as a line, and the line is a continuum of survival. Contentment and thriving is above the line, and below the line is suffering and struggle. Burnout is below the line. Every so often I dip above the line, and going below the line is regular, but mostly I'm just surviving. Because we're already carrying so much trauma and existing in such precarious environments that we can never get to a point above the line in order to experience sustainable thriving. So this means burnout is first a societal problem. Society makes us sick, it makes us unhealthy and burnout is a symptom of this. Doctors always talk about "prevention not cure" and in burnout's case, prevention would be societal change. The cure? Space to rest. The reason it's so hard to manage and navigate and recover from is because there seems to be no solution, no support systems, no hope. You recognise that the only way things can change is if society changes – but this also feels like an impossible task from the point of burnout. It's a feeling that not only am I empty, but ... Will I ever be full again? Will I ever reach a place where I can do the things that I love to do again? And it's impossible to find hope because you can't access a place to rest, recharge. That's why I think marginalised communities feel it the most.'

— *Jasmine Isa Qureshi (Queer Rootz)*

'In an embodied sense, burnout feels like a sense of heaviness and desperation. When I feel burnt out, there's a lot of frustration and hatred towards the world, the chasm between this world and the world that we all deserve to live in. There's this word called *Weltschmerz* in German that means "world-pain: a feeling of melancholy or weariness about life arising from the acute awareness of evil and suffering". So I think that burnout in a social sense is the exploitation of hope. For those of us who are putting in the effort, paying our dues or doing our community work, or activism, society manipulates that hope and that passion and that drive and takes it away from us.'

— *Aiyana Goodfellow (Neuromancers, DELINQUENTS)*

'We pathologise anything that doesn't measure up to the "good, productive, able white male" archetype, but really burnout is a quite normal, or natural result of being in a capitalist system. Despite understanding this, it's been interesting to recognise how much I've become desensitised to it. Maybe it's the harshness of life as a working-class Northerner, or of being in the charity sector, where every single person is burnt out, but I find it really hard to say I have burnout unless I'm literally bedridden. However in recent years I've been realising that I have ADHD, which has helped me see that I go through cycles of burnout, through the manic, hyperactivity, followed by jetlagged periods of having a completely empty cup. I've also started to hear Black and people of colour describing themselves as burnt out more, which has been helpful for me. Maybe it's that we're starting to believe we can claim exhaustion or be allowed to rest, you know?'

— Martha Awojobi (BAME Online)

'Burnout comes from isolation. And that isolation comes from people who are marginalised by society, being separated from a sense of community. Then that isolation causes people to be overworked, overstressed, not able to find time and space to rest, to recover, to kind of get that holistic healing that comes from the sense of community. Because we only interact with community when we need something. So I'd say burnout comes from the combination of the oppressions that we face in society and the isolation that comes from that.'

— Eshe Kiama Zuri (Co-Care)

'I think burnout is when there's an element of care being given, but it doesn't feel like that's coming back. This is the message I sent to my employer when my partner said she thought I was burnt out. I told him I didn't really understand what burnout means to me, and decided to describe how I was feeling instead: 'I don't think it's realistic for me to come into work tomorrow or this week. I'm currently exhausted and finding it daunting to leave the house, near impossible to do so for any length of time or obligation. Day-to-day requirements or low-level activity are currently overwhelming. And I find myself feeling incapacitated in relation to most of them.'

— Sim Wadiwala (Radical Routes Co-op)

'What burnout describes is disillusionment, a loss of hope. This feeling of, like, I can scream until I'm blue in the face, until they drop my body down into the earth, but it's not going to do anything. Our ancestors have been screaming "get your foot off my neck" for centuries and though there has been some change, it's been incremental and not without a fight, not without generations of us burning out from screaming and screaming and putting all our energy into this cause. We burn out from the disappointment of not being able to see an impact, of not seeing the needle move.'

— Chelsea A. Jackson (Cradle Community)

'The word that comes to me when I think of burnout is "depletion". A depletion of light, of energy, of capacity, of creativity, and also motivation. For me, this comes when my actions and values don't align. Burnout has those two movements, a tugging and pulling between the person I could be, and the person I have to be to survive. I think everyone is suffering under a capitalist system in this way. But when you are a person of colour we burn out because we're also carrying the conscious or unconscious knowing that we'll never be given the opportunity to be who we could be without violence.'

— Aurélia Saint-Just (Ulex)

'The first time I experienced burnout was 2020. I was pregnant throughout the pandemic and my son was born in the very early days of the George Floyd uprising, when our work was at an all-time high. He then got really sick, and we were worried he wouldn't survive, but the work didn't stop. I think I was running on adrenaline then. It was the year after, when I experienced this wave of what felt like crushing impossibility. My heart gave way. I'd call it a semi-heart attack, a borderline heart attack. I was twenty-nine at the time. I think from that moment I had an understanding of what my body was holding, even if I wasn't cognitively acknowledging it. It was just a spiritual exhaustion – deeper than the body. It's interesting, it wasn't until I experienced the physical and emotional severity of what burnout can cause that I realised I had never seen a Black woman rested.'

– Amahra Spence (MAIA, YARD, ABUELOS, The Black
Land and Spatial Justice Project)

'I guess where I start is from an understanding that the system is inherently extractive: the economic system was created to care for some people and not for others. Beyond that, some people are defined as a commodity. Especially Black bodies, feminised bodies, disabled bodies, queer and trans bodies. To be a commodity is to be denied the opportunity to understand your own capacity. If an awareness of your capacity doesn't really exist, then you can just be an infinite resource to the system. I think we really internalise this. A lot of Black, femme, queer people aren't able to apply the concept of boundaries, myself included. And I think a big part of burnout is that consistent neglect of your own needs and your own bodily capacity, until you just reach a kind of emptiness, I guess. The economic system means that emptiness just exists as a default for most people.'

– Noni Makuyana (Decolonising Economics)

'You have to be delusional to a degree to do this work. A combination of delusion, optimism, hope, anger, pissed-off-ness. Burnout is almost like you don't have enough energy to keep up the delusion. I remember I left an organisation a few years ago, and I was just done, spent, I had nothing left to give.

That's what burnout is. It's like a deep-rooted tiredness. Not a tiredness that can be solved by a nap, or like a good night's sleep. A multifaceted *exhaustion*. As activists, but specifically as Black women, we're so used to pushing through, to giving, giving, giving, to extending and overextending ourselves constantly, and the systems that we're working to reimagine are designed to use us to the point of burnout. There are no structures in place to hold the personal experiences that drive people to come to this work. We arrived traumatised and are retraumatised, not just by the work itself, but by the structures we're required to work within. We talk about dismantling, of tearing down walls, but it feels like constantly hitting your head against a wall that just won't break. The wall isn't breaking, but you are.'

— *Seyi Falodun-Liburd (Level Up and Project Tallawah)*

'I've got a long-standing chronic health issue so a lot of the time I do feel quite depleted, but there's a real difference between that and burnout for me, that maybe someone who hasn't lived with ill health may not understand. Tiredness is different to fatigue, but fatigue also doesn't feel like burnout. I almost imagine the fatigue is the internal — the capacities of your body. Each body might have a different level of capacity, which, when overextended could lead them to feel fatigued. Burnout then, is when that capacity is dependent on or influenced by the external. When different societal pressures and oppressions amplify that fatigue, and morph it beyond the limitations of our physical bodies. When I'm burnt out something shifts very subtly, but very importantly, in terms of how I feel within myself. It's almost like a meltdown space and saying it out loud makes me realise, it feels like a state of trauma.

A trauma response to capitalism that our bodies go into, a survival mode. There's something really perverse about it. I spend a lot of time thinking about *how do I bless this world?* But the world really isn't catered to people who have any illness or disability. It really does come back to a sense of real, psychological, spiritual, emotional lack of control. I think that's why it feels so existential to me, it's like you're being robbed of your sense of self.'

– Maymana Arefin (fungi.futures)

'We find language to articulate our experiences, and to me, "burnout" is how we articulate the ways that our body is inviting us to reset and honour its capacity. I think it's a result of sustained stress to the body and the nervous system, and a result of us being non-consensual with ourselves because of how oppression limits our choices. In capitalism, we have to work in a way that continuously forces us to be in self-abandonment. Which means our relationship to all life is one where we're in a chronic state of unsustainability and disempowerment. We're also at a time where there's so much cumulative and compounding stress; a pandemic and a climate crisis, and it's really hard to imagine a way forward. In that state of increased stress we have a smaller window of tolerance, so what we may feel or call "burnout" may actually be that we're living in a society where there is not sufficient time to reset, to regulate, to be resourced.'

– Farzana Khan (Healing Justice London)

'Burnout definitely is way more than just stress. I think that's such a disservice. Burnout for me has been a result of feeling so much pressure to protect our futures. This pressure, when within a movement, leads us to take on much more work. I think as young environmentalists we internalise a lot of external expectations that are placed on us — I know I put a lot of pressure on myself because I know what's at stake within the climate crisis, and knowing that what we do today has an impact. So many climate spaces or high-level spaces are filled with old white men, and I feel like I'm representing everyone who isn't an old white man, while not being taken seriously, while facing microaggressions because I'm not an old white man. I find these systems incredibly exhausting, especially as a young Black woman, who's neurodivergent. After COP26, for example, I ended up just not being able to speak for a while, literally forgetting how to do basic tasks. I'm usually known as the "joy/hope climate person", but burnout feels exactly like the opposite of that. It's a bit of a messy definition, but it's a messy experience.'

— Dominique Palmer

'Burnout is usually seen as a negative experience, but from a somatic perspective, the symptoms of burnout within our bodies are really red flags that our nervous system starts to wave to let us know that the way we're functioning is not okay. A variety of social conditionings have separated us from the natural connections that could regulate us, so we've become good at overriding the bodily instincts to stop, rest, or observe. That's really where I feel like our sense of collective burnout tends to stem from, this numbed disembodiment. Once we can better attune and listen to our bodies, burnout can be quite a good indicator for looking after ourselves in a way that lets us move away from racial capitalism. What's interesting is these human symptoms of burnout are replicated ecologically. Our planet's nervous system is also overheating, because we're overly impacting, extracting and over-stimulating it. Practitioners of Chinese medicine talk about bringing ourselves back to a state of harmony, and I think that's what we need for our personal and planetary health; fresh air, clean water, rest, regeneration, inaction, to be brought back to a state of harmony.'

— Kalpana Arias (Nowadays on Earth)

'I think burnout today looks very different to how burnout must have looked for our forebears. Before, burnout might have been much more around the logistics of organising in different arenas of unsafety. Now, our burnout is compounded by things like social media and "cancel culture". There's so much external and intra-community mistrust which makes everyone nervous about saying the wrong thing, doing the wrong thing, not doing enough, doing too little, being visible, not being able to make mistakes. What I imagine follows generations as a constant feature of burnout however is the insatiable need to be of service, and not knowing how to switch off from that responsibility. When you do work that is about community, and when you're involved with spaces that require a lot of sensitivity, a lot of nuance, you're constantly thinking about questions of how to make people feel safe, how to make spaces as inclusive as possible, how to constantly be as connected as possible. When those questions are always on your mind it becomes difficult to see how you and your needs fit among other people's needs.'

— Venus (Sex and Rage UK)

'Burnout's a huge topic to explore because it's connected to so many contextual paradigms across society; health, economics, environment, philanthropy, employment, colonialism, right? What we as Black and people of colour in the West – particularly the second or third generation – must reckon with are the ways we've both benefitted from and been harmed by these historical systems that are now showing up in our bodies. We see this across health justice concerns. As South Asian people, for example, we are more likely to put on weight, due to the ways our bodies adapted to starvation during the famines of colonial times. This is to say that none of this is new – burnout is just a newer way of understanding and revealing the ways that our economy is in complete conflict with the thriving of people and planet. So long as burnout isn't co-opted into something that individualises the structural conditions in which ill health is caused, we can begin to understand how our experiences are further compounded by how we are marginalised.'

– Immy Kaur (Civic Square)

'I'm from a generation – the "snowflake" generation, they call us – where it was taboo to talk about mental health, emotional health. Especially in immigrant households within sixties, seventies, eighties, even nineties Britain, we were told "no pain, no gain", and any weakness could make you unworthy of citizenship. So while burnout is really a new term for me, the feeling is something I know well, and it's nice to have a term to describe it. Because even though it sounds literal, this is exactly how it feels – like you're a match that somebody's just blown out. All your light, your energy, your life force has been completely extinguished and you're just left in your own heavy, veiled darkness, with nothing else to give.'

– Ola Fagbohun (The Zest OF: You Project)

'Burnout to me is:

A symptom of a root problem that our bodies have been screaming at us to listen to. It's telling us that our physical, mental and spiritual systems are collapsing. Yet we ignore its cries of exhaustion because we live in a system where our rest is commodified.

A somatic response to becoming unseasonable. The harm we inflict on nature is a reflection of what we're doing to ourselves.

A fear of falling asleep, because the thought of waking up and facing the next day is unbearable.

A navigation, constantly assessing if a place is safe. Then, an acceptance — this world isn't accessible for us.

A losing-sight of the really pure and loving parts of being alive: energy, and imagination, the ability to dream into the future and create new worlds.

An inability to meet the basic needs we require to live a healthy, safe, loving life.

A confinement. Where my bed, which should be a safe place, becomes the prison that I am bound to for eight months at a time.

An acknowledgement — that if we don't choose rest days, our bodies will choose them for us.

A bureaucratic nightmare. Of navigating soulless government systems like the HMRC and the DWP.

A darkening — in losing connection with friends and letting go of passions which gave us light.

A battleground where every day becomes a warzone.

A loneliness we never knew was even possible.

A constant calculation. *If I shower today, will I have the energy to eat?*

An erasure, as the tiny pencil drawing of the person we once were is forgotten.

An anger. Pure unfiltered rage.

A permission – to rest, to slow down, to be held, to ask for help.

An inability to know what our needs are until they have – or haven't – been met.

An open invitation, recognising we need each other, and that we are codependent on the care of others.

A learning of very important life lessons, such as: *there is no honour in self-sacrifice.*

A constant FOMO, of our bodies not being able to gift our brains the drinks with friends or spontaneous outings that they crave.

A burdening. Like wearing armour that has moulded to our skin. It's rusted, heavy, weighing us down but we can't detach from it. Maybe it protected us once, but not any more.

A coldness – of needing the warmth of the sun on our face or the touch of a human embrace that reassures us that everything's going to be okay.

A lot of days, months, years spent mourning and grieving what could have been. Attending a lot of funerals for ourselves.

I wonder, honestly, if anyone who has never experienced the exhaustions and traumas of such systems – the racism and ableism of racial capitalism – can ever conceptualise, never mind experience, burnout.'

– Azekel Axelle (The Black Trans Foundation)

Gratitudes

When I began writing *Radical Rest*, I had a vision for what the process would look like: a whimsical, romantic, nature-fuelled self-actualisation. It's safe to say that the reality did not live up to my Beatrix Potter fantasy, and I have learned the hard way that for working-class writers of colour like myself, it rarely ever does.

At scarily regular intervals during this writing process, I have wondered if what this book could possibly give the world will ever be worth what it's taken from me, required of me, in order to write it. In my more glass-half-full reflections, however, I can see that this journey has ultimately gifted me the one thing that consistently makes the artist's plight feel worthwhile: love.

In the moments where I couldn't love or be kind to myself, the love and kindness I have received from others has been overwhelming. Those who were present and astute to my shifting capacities, who let me show up in my vulnerabilities, communicate my needs and then met them by simply posing 'how can we help?' This support was not grandiose or extravagant, yet I noticed every quiet, subtle act which told me it was okay to pause being in service of others, so that I could embrace being taken care of.

These offerings reminded me that love comes in so many forms. It looks like screaming from the precipice of a Peak District edge, being taken to nervous-system-resetting saunas, the *clink clink* of spicy margaritas toasting the success of making it through another week, homemade meals delivered in Tupperware boxes, spare rooms, allotment sheds, outhouses, baths and bedrooms offered as makeshift office spaces, snuggles on demand (both human and feline) and joyful routines – midday walks and monthly swims which equated to a monumental provision: something to look forward to, something to live for.

A woefully neglected houseplant feels like a good analogy for who I have become during the past two years, and yet *Radical Rest* has sprouted, a resilient bud blooming despite it all. To the people who provided a nutrient-rich earth in which the seeds of this book could be planted: my mum, Diane; my brother, Keith; my favourite person, Sam; my inspiration, Mary; my family, Bradley, Alice, Christie.

To those who offered support and mentorship when *Radical Rest* was but a seedling: L'Oreal, Shahed, Charlie, Black Girl Writers, Megan, Mireille, Abi and The Good Literary Agency.

To my interviewees, whose wisdoms and insights directed me towards the sun: Aiyana, Amahra, Aurélia, Azekel, Chelsea, Dominique, Eshe, Farzana, Immy, Jasmine, Kalpana, Kavian, Martha, Maymana, Noni, Ola, Seyi, Sim, Venus and Vera. Plus, those who were not featured in these pages, but whose contributions were foundational to its growth: Abdi, Dwight, Jumoke, Yasin.

To the organisational spaces that watered me, revived me, when I began to wither: RESOLVE Collective, Decolonising Economics, Migration Matters Festival, MAIA, Healing Justice London and so many more.

To the practitioners whose treatments and therapies have routinely kept me firmly planted, grounded, and held upright: Vanessa, Rainy, Muna, Eddie and all at Dharnakosa.

To those who facilitated writing workshops that helped me tend to my growth, even at its unruliest: Arvon, Written into Being, Midnight and Indigo, Our True Nature, Rutgers' Poets and Scholars Summer Retreat.

To Shropshire, Somerset, Cambridge, North Wales, the Scottish Highlands, the Yorkshire Dales, and my beloved Peak District – the environments which formed a boundless backdrop to the writing process; and to those who opened their homes to me throughout: Dal, Lou at Flying Horse Lawn, Hafsah and David, Bradley, Lindsey and Amos, Val and Jo.

To the institutions that have financially resourced me in times of scarcity: Society of Authors, Sheffield Writers Development Grant, the Journalists' Charity.

And to those who helped me harvest the crop that you hold in your hands today: Sarah, Amy, Sabrena, Megan, Pippa and the Dark Matter Agency.

For once, I am lost for words.

Just eternally grateful.

Notes

Notes on Language

1. M. Jones, "'If Black Women Were Free': An Oral History of the Combahee River Collective', *The Nation* (29 October 2021); https://www.thenation.com/article/society/combahee-river-collective-oral-history/
2. S. Faye, *The Transgender Issue* (London: Penguin Random House, 2021), p. xiii
3. L. Olufemi, *Experiments in Imagining Otherwise* (London: Hajar Press, 2021), p. 3
4. S. Manzoor-Khan, *Seeing for Ourselves and Even Stranger Possibilities* (London: Hajar Press, 2023), p. 65

Introduction

1. O. E. Butler, *Parable of the Talents* (London: Headline Publishing Group, 1998), p. 129
2. ibid., p. 127
3. ibid., p. 121
4. ibid., p. 52
5. H. Jovanovic et al., 'Chronic stress is linked to 5-HT(1A) receptor changes and functional disintegration of the limbic networks', *Neuroimage*, vol. 55 (2011), pp. 1178–88
6. I. Savic, 'Structural changes of the brain in relation to occupational stress', *CerebCortex*, 18 December 2013 [Epub ahead of print]
7. C. Liston et al., 'Psychosocial stress reversibly disrupts prefrontal processing and attentional control', *Proceedings of the National Academy of Sciences*, 106 (2009); pp. 912–7; doi:10.1073/pnas.0807041106
8. E. Blix et al., 'Long-Term Occupational Stress Is Associated with Regional Reductions in Brain Tissue Volumes', *PLoS ONE vol.* 8, no. 6, e64065 (2013); doi:10.1371/journal.pone.0064065
9. B. G. Oosterholt et al., 'Burnout and cortisol: Evidence for a lower cortisol awakening response in both clinical and nonclinical burnout', *Journal of Psychosomatic Research*, vol. 78, no. 5 (2015), pp. 445–51; doi:10.1016/j.jpsychores.2014.11.003
10. R. W. Gilmore, 'Making Abolition Geography in California's Central Valley', *The Funambulist* (20 December 2018); https://thefunambulist

.net/magazine/21-space-activism/interview-making-abolition-geography-california-central-valley-ruth-wilson-gilmore

11. N. White et al, 'Effective Activist: An Evidence-Based guide to Progressive Social Change', *Effective Activist Zine* (date unknown); https://effective activist.com/

12. Unknown, 'A Litany for Survival: The Life and Work of Audre Lorde', *Bomb* (1 July 1996); https://bombmagazine.org/articles/1996/07/01/a-litany-for-survival-the-life-and-work-of-audre-lorde/; A. Gay Griffin, M. Parkerson (directors), 'A Litany for Survival: The Life and Work of Audre Lorde' (1995), A Third World Newsreel production

13. D. Iyer, *The Social Change Map*, 2017; https://www.socialchangemap.com/home/understanding-the-framework

14. b. hooks, *Teaching to Transgress* (New York: Routledge, 1994), p. 74

15. 'Geographies of Racial Capitalism with Ruth Wilson Gilmore – An Antipode Foundation film', YouTube (1 June 2020); https://www.youtube.com/watch?v=2CS627aKrJI

On Radical Exhaustion

1. M. Kaba, 'So You're Thinking About Becoming an Abolitionist', LEVEL (30 October 2020); https://level.medium.com/so-youre-thinking-about-becoming-an-abolitionist-a436f8e31894

2. R. Ellison, 'Richard Wright's Blues', in *Shadow and Act* (New York: Signet Books, 1966), p. 90

3. '"Blue Monday" artist Annie Lee, dead at 79', *Chicago Tribune* (26 November 2014); https://www.chicagotribune.com/entertainment/ct-artist-annie-lee-dead-at-79-20141126-column.html

4. D. Inman, 'Lizzo Recreates "Blue Monday" painting during "Saturday Night Live" Performance', *VIBE* (19 December 2022); https://www.vibe.com/news/movies-tv/lizzo-blue-monday-snl-performance-1234720259/

5. 'righteous mind', YouTube (16 July 2012); https://www.youtube.com/watch?v=HkeqIXPmLIc

6. F. Douglass, *My Bondage and Freedom* (New Haven, CT: Yale University Press, 2014), p. 79

7. B. Resnick, 'The Racial Inequality of Sleep', *The Atlantic* (27 October 2015); https://www.theatlantic.com/health/archive/2015/10/the-sleep-gap-and-racial-inequality/412405/

8. A. Blackwelder, M. Hoskins, L. Huber, 'Effect of Inadequate Sleep on Frequent Mental Distress', *Prev Chronic Dis* (2021); 18:200573. DOI: http://dx.doi.org/10.5888/pcd18.200573

9. 'Insomnia', *NHS Inform* (3 May 2023); https://www.nhsinform.scot/illnesses-and-conditions/mental-health/insomnia#:~:text=Insomnia%20is%20

difficulty%20getting%20to,particularly%20common%20in%20elderly%20 people

10. J. Clarabut, 'Are You Getting Enough Quality Sleep?', *Wellbeing People* (24 November 2023); https://www.wellbeingpeople.com/2020/03/10/ are-you-getting-enough-quality-sleep/

11. L. Bent, 'Women lose three hours sleep a night because of their partners', *iNews* (8 October 2020); https://inews.co.uk/inews-lifestyle/women-lose-sleep-night-because-partners-319075

12. R. Moss, 'Almost Half of British Women are Sleep Deprived and Risking Long-Term Health Effects, Report Warns', *Huffington Post* (26 January 2016); https://www.huffingtonpost.co.uk/2016/01/26/half-of-women-in-uk-sleep-deprived_n_9076030.html

13. C. Joseph, 'Eternally Woke: Why aren't Black women getting enough sleep?', *gal-dem* (21 January 2020); https://gal-dem.com/eternally-woke-why-arent-black-women-getting-enough-sleep

14. R. Newsom and K. Truong, 'Sleep Apnea and Heart Disease', *Sleep Foundation* (15 June 2023); https://www.sleepfoundation.org/sleep-apnea/sleep-apnea-linked-heart-disease#:~:text=It's%20estimated%20that%20patients%20 with,coronary%20heart%20disease%20by%2030%25

15. Bare Minimum Collective, 'The Bare Minimum Manifesto' (6 March 2020); https://medium.com/@bareminimum/the-bare-minimum-manifesto-bfedbbc9dd71

16. 'The Last Breath Society (Coughing Coffin)', Institute of Contemporary Arts; https://www.ica.art/live/the-last-breath-society-coughing-coffin-2021#:~:text=Martin%20O'Brien%20was%20born,living%20in%20 'zombie%20time'

17. R. Wilson Gilmore, *Abolition Geography* (London: Verso, 2022), p. 107

18. M. Mariani, 'The Tragic, Forgotten History of Zombies', *The Atlantic* (28 October, 2015); https://www.theatlantic.com/entertainment/archive/2015/10/how-america-erased-the-tragic-history-of-the-zombie/412264/

19. A. Mbembe, 'Necropolitics', *Public Culture*, vol. 15, no. 1 (2003), pp. 11–40, p. 17

20. ibid., p. 27

21. ibid., 40

22. 'Tricia Hersey: Rest & Collective Care as Tools for Liberation', YouTube (9 April 2021); https://www.youtube.com/watch?v=7OuXnLrKyi0

23. T. Hersey, *Rest as Resistance* (London: Hachette, 2022)

24. ibid., p. 96

25. ibid., p. 97

Case Study #1: The Home

1. b. hooks, *Yearning: Race, Gender, and Cultural Politics* (New York: Routledge, 2014), p. 61

2. F. Vergès, *A Feminist Theory of Violence* (London: Pluto Press, 2022), p. 4

3. INCITE!, *The Revolution Will Not Be Funded: Beyond the Non-Profit Industrial Complex* (Durham, NC: Duke University Press, 2017)

4. 'Progress on the Sustainable Development Goals: The Gender Snapshot 2023', United Nations; https://www.unwomen.org/sites/default/files/2023-09/progress-on-the-sustainable-development-goals-the-gender-snapshot-2023-en.pdf

5. 'Women Shoulder the Responsibility of "Unpaid Work"', ONS (10 November 2016); https://www.ons.gov.uk/employmentandlabourmarket/people inwork/earningsandworkinghours/articles/womenshouldertheresponsibilityofunpaidwork/2016-11-10

6. P. H. Collins, 'It's all in the family: Intersections of Gender, Race, and Nation', *Hypatia*, Vol. 13, No. 3 (1998), pp. 62–82; https://www.jstor.org/stable/3810699?read-now=1&oauth_data=eyJlbWFpbCI6InBlYWtzb2Zjb2xvdXJhZ21haWwuY29tIiwiW5zdGl0dXRpb25JZHHMiOltdLCJwcm92aWRlcilI6Imdvb2dsZSJ9#page_scan_tab_contents

7. Cradle Community, *Brick by Brick: How We Build a World Without Prisons* (London: Hajar Press, 2021), p. 62

8. N. Calcea, 'Rent prices: How much have they gone up in your area?', *BBC News* (29 March 2023); https://www.bbc.co.uk/news/business-65103937

9. Cradle Community, *Brick by Brick*, pp. 62–3

10. The Care Collective, *The Care Manifesto* (London: Versus, 2020), p. 6

On Radical Grief

1. @ash-s0ul, TikTok, 8 August 2022; https://www.tiktok.com/@ashs0ul/video/7129325858132856110?_t=8k6G3TBNxfl&_r=1; T. Dixon (director); 'Meeting The Man: James Baldwin in Paris' (1970)

2. @alokvmenon, Instagram, 20 March 2024; https://www.instagram.com/reel/C4t7QCiuKqi/?igsh=MThxMHZleWl0OXJueg==

3. N. Vaswani, 'Bereavement among young men in Prison', *Criminal Justice Matters*, vol. 98 (2014); https://www.crimeandjustice.org.uk/publications/cjm/article/bereavement-among-young-men-prison

4. G. Bhattacharyya, *We, the Heartbroken* (London: Hajar Press, 2023), p. 4

5. Various contributors, 'Life-Affirming Infrastructures' [panel conversation], Healing Justice London (2023); https://healingjusticeldn.org/resources/life-affirming-infrastructures/

6. O. Moshfegh, *My Year of Rest and Relaxation* (London: Penguin Random House, 2018), p. 51

7. @co_cu1tur3, Instagram post, 25th November 2023; https://www.instagram. com/reel/Cz-0XMKRZh8/?igshid=MzRlODBiNWFlZA==

8. D. Kular, 'Our Wild Cemetery Writing Tips' (2023)

9. R. Wall Kimmerer, *Braiding Sweetgrass* (London: Penguin Random House, 2020), p. 17

10. Bhattacharyya, *We, the Heartbroken*, p. 4

11. ibid., p. 8

12. E. Muir, 'Building a Home for Grief in Edale', *Slow Ways* (16 May 2023); https://stories.slowways.org/building-a-home-for-grief-in-edale/

13. Bhattacharyya, *We, the Heartbroken*, p. 115

On Radical Rage

1. 'D. Stewart, 'Black Rage in an Anti-Black World Is a Spiritual Virtue', *Sojourners* (29 May 2020); https://sojo.net/articles/black-rage-anti-black-world-spiritual-virtue

2. A. Lorde, *Sister Outsider* (Berkeley, CA: Crossing Press, 1984), p. 129

3. 'Getting the balance right? An inspection of how effectively the police deal with protests', HMICFRS report (2021); https://hmicfrs.justiceinspectorates. gov.uk/publications/getting-the-balance-right-an-inspection-of-how-effectively-the-police-deal-with-protests/

4. 'Solange performing Mad at Lovebox 2017', YouTube (15 July 2017); https:// www.youtube.com/watch?v=-72Vxurbld8

5. L. R. Owens, *Love and Rage: The Path of Liberation Through Anger* (Berkeley, CA: North Atlantic Books, 2020), p. 69

6. ibid., p. 75

7. 'Stephanie Jones-Rogers, "they were her property white women as slave owners in the American South"', YouTube (5 March 2021); https://www. youtube.com/watch?v=BTOv3uitsh0&t=1550s

8. R. Hamad, *White Tears/Brown Scars: How White Feminism Betrays Women of Color* (London: Trapeze, 2020), p. 86

9. 'Amy Cooper Made 2nd Call To 911 About Black Birdwatcher, Prosecutors Say', YouTube (15 October 2020); https://www.youtube.com/watch?v= L3662COVmn8&t=99s

10. E. Muir, 'How can we end gendered violence, when the Violence Against Women and Girls sector is violent?', *gal-dem* (9 June 2022); https://gal-dem. com/gendered-violence-vawg-sector/

Case Study #2: Education

1. P. Freire, *Pedagogy of the Oppressed* (New York, NY: Continuum, 2000) p. 34

2. UCLA School of Critical Race Studies, 'CRT Forward: Tracking the Attack on Critical Race Theory' (2023); https://crtforward.law.ucla.edu/wp-content/uploads/2023/04/UCLA-Law_CRT-Report_Final.pdf

3. R. Merrick, 'Schools minister rejects lessons about colonialism, and slave trade in case they "lower standards"', *The Independent* (25 February 2021); https://www.independent.co.uk/news/uk/politics/school-compulsory-lessons-colony-slave-trade-b1807571.html

4. A. Hill, 'Raising UK state pension age to 71 would bring "misery" to millions', *Guardian* (Friday 9 February 2024); https://www.theguardian.com/money/2024/feb/09/raising-uk-state-pension age

5. J. Cribb and I. O'Brien, 'Latest increase in state pension age from 65 to 66 led to income poverty rates among 65-year-olds more than doubling', *The Institute for Fiscal Studies* (20 June 2022); https://ifs.org.uk/news/latest-increase-state-pension-age-65-66-led-income-poverty-rates-among-65-year-olds-more

6. Freire, *Pedagogy of the Oppressed*, p. 46

7. A. Davis, 'Over 75% of students have experienced stress or anxiety, over exam changes, research reveals', *The Standard* (25 February 2021); https://www.standard.co.uk/news/education/75-percent-students-stress-anxiety-exam-changes-research-b921049.html

8. b. hooks, *Teaching to Transgress* (New York, NY: Routledge, 1994), p. 61

9. S. Bateman, 'Updated: Doncaster school excludes pupils more often than any other in England', *Doncaster Free Press* (16 September 2022); https://www.doncasterfreepress.co.uk/education/updated-doncaster-school-excludes-pupils-more-often-than-any-other-in-england-3844093

10. hooks, *Teaching to Transgress*, pp. 69–70

11. ibid., p. 15

12. Freire, *Pedagogy of the Oppressed*, p. 22

13. E. Fromm, *The Heart of Man* (New York, NY: 1966), p. 52–3, quoted in Freire, *Pedagogy of the Oppressed*, p. 22

14. S. Mitchell, *Sacred Instructions* (Berkeley, CA: North Atlantic Books, 2018), p. 213

15. ibid., p. 11

16. ibid., p. 210

On Radical Anxiety

1. A. Khan, 'Capitalism overwhelms our senses while also insulating us from the connection we need', *Cosmic Anarchy* (31 March 2023); https://wokescientist.substack.com/p/capitalism-overwhelms-our-senses

2. I. Umebinyuo, *Questions for Ada* (Scotts Valley, CA: CreateSpace, 2015), p. 79

3. T. Tsui, *It's Not Just You: How to Navigate Eco-Anxiety and the Climate Crisis* (London: Simon & Schuster, 2023), p. 13

4. @OurResilienceProject, Instagram post, 10 July 2023: https://www. instagram.com/p/CuhSVHgt9LK/?img_index=1

On Radical Abundance

1. J. Odell, *Saving Time: Discovering a Life Beyond the Clock* (London: Penguin Random House, 2023), p. 238

2. D. Pegg, R. Evans and S. Carrell, 'King Charles to receive huge pay rise from UK taxpayers', *Guardian* (20 July 2023); https://www. theguardian.com/uk-news/2023/jul/20/king-charles-to-receive-huge-pay-rise-from-uk-taxpayers

3. P. Crerar, 'Keir Starmer defends decision not to scrap two-child benefit cap', *Guardian* (18 July 2023); https://www.theguardian.com/politics/2023/jul/18/keir-starmer-defends-decision-not-to-scrap-two-child-benefit-cap

4. H. Bancroft, 'Almost 5,000 more deaths due to cold homes as Treasury fails to give out £440m in energy support', *Independent* (6 September 2023); https://www.independent.co.uk/news/uk/home-news/winter-deaths-cold-homes-energy-support-b2406316.html

5. 'More than a third of workers in the UK consider changing jobs to combat the rising cost of living', *Totaljobs* (9 March 2022); https://www.totaljobs.com/media-centre/more-than-a-third-of-workers-in-the-uk-consider-changing-jobs-to-combat-the-rising-cost-of-living

6. 'CHAIN Statistics: Cost of living homelessness crisis', *Salvation Army* (31 January 2023); https://www.salvationarmy.org.uk/news/chain-statistics-cost-living-homelessness-crisis#:~:text=This%20is%20a%2021%25%20increase,cost%20of%20living%20to%20spiral

7. 'Who We Are', Cooperation Jackson; https://cooperationjackson.org/intro

8. 'About', Decolonising Economics; https://decolonisingeconomics.org/about/

9. 'Full spectrum community care', Eshe Kiama Zuri; https://eshekiamazuri.com/fscc

Case Study #3: The Charity Industrial Complex

1. M. Kaba, 'Free Us All', *The New Inquiry* (8 May 2017); https://thenewinquiry.com/free-us-all/

2. 'How many charities are there?', How Charities Work; https://howcharitieswork.com/about-charities/how-many-charities/

3. ibid.

4. A. Ricketts, 'Nine in 10 charity workers have felt stress, overwhelm or burnout over the past year, survey shows', *ThirdSector* (20 January 2021); https://www.thirdsector.co.uk/nine-10-charity-workers-felt-stress-overwhelm-burnout-past-year-survey-shows/management/article/1705083

5. INCITE!, *The Revolution Will Not Be Funded: Beyond the Non-Profit Industrial Complex* (Durham, NC: Duke University Press, 2017), p. 8

6. The Trussell Trust, 'Emergency Food Parcel Distribution in the UK: April 2022–March 2023'; https://www.trusselltrust.org/wp-content/uploads/sites/2/2023/04/EYS-UK-Factsheet-2022-23.pdf

7. Cradle Community, *Brick by Brick: How We Build a World Without Prisons* (London: Hajar Press, 2021), p. 54

8. ibid., p. 117

9. L. Scarman, *The Scarman Report: The Brixton Disorders 10–12 April 1981* (Middlesex: Penguin, 1986), p. 209

10. ibid., p. xiii

11. A. Shafi and I. Nagdee, *Race to the Bottom: Reclaiming Antiracism* (London: Pluto Press, 2022), pp. 76–7

12. A. S. Day and S. O. McBean, *Abolition Revolution* (London: Pluto Press, 2022), p. 19

13. ibid., pp. 19–20

14. ibid., p. 19

15. INCITE!, *The Revolution Will Not Be Funded*, p. xxi

On Radical Joy

1. a. m. brown, *Pleasure Activism: The Politics of Feeling Good* (Chico, CA: AK Press, 2019), p. 12

2. 'AISHA PARIS SMITH: Pleasure is a necessity: resourcing our bodies with joy', YouTube (22 June 2023); https://www.youtube.com/watch?v=bAYzfBbbMBw

3. 'Audre Lorde reads Uses of the Erotic: The Erotic As Power (FULL Updated)', YouTube (2 August 2019); https://www.youtube.com/watch?v=aWmq9gw4Rq0; originally a paper presented at the Fourth Berkshire Conference on the History of Women, Mount Holyoke College, 25 August, 1978

4. ibid.

5. C. Brinkhurst-Cuff and T. Sotire (eds), *Black Joy* (London: Penguin Random House, 2021), p. 72

6. ibid., p. 77

7. brown, *Pleasure Activism*, p. 13

8. 'Audre Lorde reads Uses of the Erotic', YouTube

9. A. P. Smith, 'Joy and The Body' [course], hosted on Advaya; https://advaya.co/events/2023/08/15/joy-and-the-body-an-online-course-with-aisha-paris-smith

10. 'Audre Lorde reads Uses of the Erotic', YouTube

11. E. Muir, 'The Show Must Go On: The Reinvention of Migration Matters Festival', *Corridor8* (2 July 2020); https://corridor8.co.uk/article/the-show-must-go-on-the-reinvention-of-migration-matters-festival/

12. ibid.
13. 'Audre Lorde reads Uses of the Erotic', YouTube
14. 'Transcript: In conversation with Ruth Wilson Gilmore', UCL (7 June 2020); https://www.ucl.ac.uk/racism-racialisation/transcript-conversation-ruth-wilson-gilmore
15. 'Pastoral Interludes', V&A Collections; https://collections.vam.ac.uk/item/O107865/pastoral-interludeits-as-if-the-photograph-pollard-ingrid/
16. A. Ghadiali, '"People want me to say I'm alienated": Ingrid Pollard on the myths of art, race and landscape', *Guardian* (20 March 2020); https://www.theguardian.com/artanddesign/2022/mar/20/ingrid-pollard-myths-art-race-landscape-photography-interview-mk-gallery

On Radical Hope

1. A. V. Morales 'V'ahavta' (25 July 2016); http://www.auroralevinsmorales.com/blog/vahavta
2. C. A. Jackson, 'Post-Charity Burnout w/ Evie Muir', *Post-Woke Podcast* (February 2023); https://open.spotify.com/episode/0mG845iF2f6uXhTTIrNalK
3. K. Salaam, 'History: Octavia Butler Gave Us A Few Rules For Predicting The Future', *Neo-Griot* (2020); https://kalamu.com/neogriot/2013/07/09/history-octavia-butler-gave-us-a-few-rules-for-predicting-the-future/
4. L. Olufemi, *Experiments in Imagining Otherwise* (London: Hajar Press, 2021), pp. 11–12
5. T. Campt, *Listening to Images* (Durham, NC: Duke University Press, 2017), p. 17
6. Olufemi, *Experiments in Imagining Otherwise*, p. 7
7. ibid., p. 35
8. '(Pt 15) Under the Blacklight: Storytelling While Black and Female: Conjuring Beautiful Experiments', YouTube (6 August 2020); https://www.youtube.com/watch?v=xGS5aP5Vi7g
9. M. Arefin, 'Mapping Alternative Futures through Fungi: The Usefulness of Mycorrhizal Networks as a Metaphor for Mutual Aid', *UCL/Research Gate* (15 September 2021): https://www.researchgate.net/publication/359294856_Mapping_Alternative_Futures_through_Fungi_The_Usefulness_of_Mycorrhizal_Networks_as_a_Metaphor_for_Mutual_Aid
10. A. Emejulu, *Fugitive Feminism* (London: Silver Press, 2022), p. 23
11. ibid., p. 9
12. ibid.
13. ibid., p. 30

Case Study #4: The Health Sector

1. Bare Minimum Collective, 'The Bare Minimum Manifesto' (6 March 2020); https://medium.com/@bareminimum/the-bare-minimum-manifesto-bfedbbc9dd71

2. Stonewall, 'School Report' (June 2017); https://www.stonewall.org.uk/school-report-2017

3. B. Alder-Bolton and A. Vierkant, *Health Communism* (London: Verso, 2022), p. xiv

4. S. Gregory, 'Sheffielders vastly more likely to be unwell and out of work compared to residents of west Oxfordshire', *Now Then Magazine* (8 February, 2024); https://nowthenmagazine.com/articles/sheffielders-vastly-more-likely-to-be-unwell-and-out-of-work-compared-to-residents-of-west-oxfordshire-inequality

5. Alder-Bolton and Vierkant, *Health Communism*, p. xiv

6. R. W. Gilmore, *Abolition Geography* (London: Verso, 2022), pp. 304–5

7. A. Sowemimo, *Divided: Racism, Medicine and Why We Need to Decolonise Healthcare* (London: Profile Books, 2023), pp. 26–7

8. ibid., p. 40

9. ibid., p. 49

10. NHS Digital, 'Ethnicity facts and figures: Psychotic disorders' (5 March 2021); www.ethnicity-facts-figures.service.gov.uk/health/mental-health/adults-experiencing-a-psychotic-disorder/latest

11. P. Fearon, J. Kirkbride, C. Morgan et al., 'Incidence of schizophrenia and other psychoses in ethnic minority groups: results from the MRC AESOP Study', *Psychol Med*, vol. 36, no. 11 (2006), pp. 1541–50

12. M. Frazer-Carroll, *Mad World: The Politics of Mental Health* (London: Pluto Press, 2023), p. 57

13. A. Y. Davis, *Are Prisons Obsolete?* (New York, NY: Seven Stories Press, 2003), p. 66

14. @cpabolition, Instagram post, 6 July 2022; https://www.instagram.com/p/CfrJ6giIp__/?hl=en&img_index=1

15. Gilmore, *Abolition Geography*, p. 359

On Radical Rest

1. Elizabeth-Jane Burnett, *The Grassling* (London: Allen Lane, 2020), p. 187

2. O. E. Butler, *Parable of the Sower* (London: Headline Publishing Group, 1993), p. 49

3. D. Nieto, 'Daily death rate in Gaza higher than any other major 21st Century conflict – Oxfam', *Oxfam* (11 January 2024); https://www.oxfam.org/en/press-releases/daily-death-rate-gaza-higher-any-other-major-21st-century-conflict-oxfam

4.   Niels de Hoog, Antonio Voce, Elena Morresi, Manisha Ganguly and Ashley Kirk, 'How war destroyed Gaza's neighbourhoods – visual investigation', *Guardian* (30 January 2024); https://www.theguardian.com/world/ng-interactive/2024/jan/30/how-war-destroyed-gazas-neighbourhoods-visual-investigation. Kaamil Ahmed, 'Lack of clean drinking water for 95% of people in Gaza threatens health crisis', *Guardian* (4 November 2023); https://www.theguardian.com/global-development/2023/nov/04/lack-of-clean-drinking-water-for-95-of-people-in-gaza-threatens-health-crisis

5.   F. Fanon, *Wretched of the Earth* (London: Penguin Classics, 2001), p. 44

6.   'The tree hugger: Settler attacks on Palestinian farmers and their olive trees | Al Jazeera World', YouTube (23 November 2023); https://www.youtube.com/watch?v=fslr2bZs864

7.   ibid.

8.   Her Farm; https://herfarmnepal.org/

9.   'Navild Acosta and Fannie Sosa Present at the 2019 Creative Capital Artist Retreat', YouTube (30 September 2019); https://www.youtube.com/watch?v=A8e672KisU8

10.   'Access to Nature in the English Countryside', CPRE (August 2021); https://www.cpre.org.uk/wp-content/uploads/2021/08/August-2021_Access-to-nature-in-the-English-countryside_research-overview.pdf

11.   Dr S. Huxtable et al, 'Interim Report on the Connections between Colonialism and Properties now in the Care of the National Trust, Including Links with Historic Slavery', *National Trust* (September 2020); https://nt.global.ssl.fastly.net/binaries/content/assets/website/national/pdf/colonialism-and-historic-slavery-report.pdf

12.   D. Letenyei, 'How much land does the Royal Family own in the World?' *Market Realist* (16 September 2022); https://marketrealist.com/global-politics/how-much-land-does-the-royal-family-own-in-the-world/

13.   'Navild Acosta and Fannie Sosa Present', YouTube

14.   Butler, *Parable of the Sower*, p. 49

15.   ibid., p. 61

16.   'Radical Self Care: Angela Davis', YouTube (17 December 2018); https://www.youtube.com/watch?v=Q1cHoL4vaBs

17.   B. Baker, 'Why I Became an Abolitionist', *Harper's Bazaar* (10 December 2020); https://www.harpersbazaar.com/culture/politics/a34473938/why-i-became-an-abolitionist/

Glossary of Re-definitions

1.   T. Morrison, *Beloved* (London: Vintage, 2007), p. 225